Men's Fitness®

TOTAL BODY PLAN

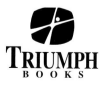

TRIUMPH
BOOKS

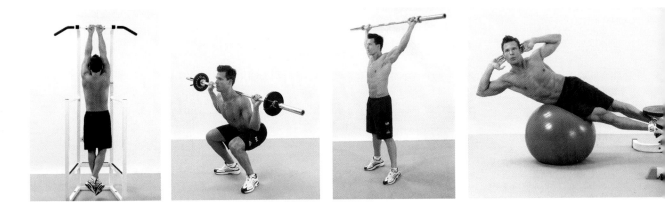

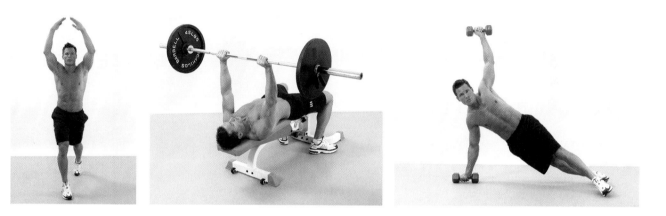

Bill Hartman is a sports performance coach, physical therapist and former competitive bodybuilder. He holds a bachelor of science degree in movement and sports science from Purdue University, where he graduated with distinction. Hartman is certified by the National Strength and Conditioning Association as a Certified Strength and Conditioning Specialist (C.S.C.S.) and with USA Weightlifting as a Sports Performance Coach. He also sits on the board of directors of the International Youth Conditioning Association. Hartman and his wife, Diane, currently reside in Indianapolis, Indiana.

Adam Campbell, C.S.C.S., is the Fitness Editor for *Men's Fitness*. He holds a master's degree in exercise physiology from the University of Kansas, where he worked as an assistant researcher for two years in the human performance and weight loss laboratories. He is also the co-author of the *Testosterone Advantage Plan*. Campbell and his girlfriend, Jessica, live with their three dogs in Allentown, Pennsylvania.

Library of Congress Control Number: 2006938706

This book is available in quantity at special discounts for your group or organization. For further information, contact:

Triumph Books
542 South Dearborn Street
Suite 750
Chicago, Illinois 60605
(312) 939-3330
Fax (312) 663-3557

Printed in U.S.A.
ISBN: 978-1-57243-971-9

Table of Contents

As the Fitness Editor of *Men's Fitness*® magazine, I receive thousands of letters, phone calls and e-mails from our readers every year. Some are story ideas, some are thank you's and a few are … not so pleasant. But the majority by far are questions. And they're almost all some version of one very simple question: "How do I gain muscle and lose fat?" Unfortunately, the answer isn't so simple.

Simultaneously gaining muscle while losing fat is a physiological paradox. You'll have a hard time doing it since the faster you gain muscle, the harder it is for your body to shed fat, and vice versa. A more effective approach is to do each separately. Most guys refer to this as "bulking" and "cutting." That is, you do a bulking phase to add maximum muscle size, followed by a cutting phase to lose fat and become as lean as possible.

Of course, tell a guy to bulk first and then cut and you create an entirely new set of questions, starting with, "How do I do that?" And unless a complete answer is given, every response just generates more questions. The only place to start is at the beginning. And that's why we created this book.

Fortunately, my job gives me access to the top fitness experts in the world. So finding a great strength coach to design the training plans in this book wasn't a problem. The trick was finding the *right* strength coach. I wanted to give you, the readers, the ultimate solution for sculpting a lean, muscular body. It had to be simple. It had to be original. And it had to be more effective than any plan I'd ever seen. But that was no easy task.

Although I'm exposed to new training ideas on a daily basis, most of them are unoriginal and worthless, especially the ones promoted by celebrities and infomercials. Of the few that are effective, even fewer are innovative.

Luckily, I found Bill Hartman. He had posted a string of replies on a fitness message board that I frequent. The questions that he answered were basic; the answers weren't. In fact, most of them surprised me. He used concepts that were entirely new to me and I could immediately tell that Bill was on a completely different level than 99 percent of the strength coaches I'd ever met. A few conversations later and we were writing this book together. Besides being an expert strength coach, Bill is also a physical therapist. This allows him to create training programs that aren't just effective for building muscle and losing fat, but that are also designed to prevent and reduce the risk of injuries. That keeps you in the gym and off the disabled list, ensuring that you're continually improving your body.

Our goal wasn't to re-invent the wheel. We simply wanted to take the basic training principles that we know work and tweak them to create a smarter, more efficient plan. Most importantly, though, we wanted you to be able to customize it for your body, a feature that's missing from all of the other one-size-fits-all workout programs.

Few guys – even top fitness experts – ever learn the concepts presented in this book. So if you're a beginner, consider yourself lucky. You'll be far ahead of the game from the get-go and that translates into quick increases in muscle size and strength. If you're an experienced lifter, be prepared to make the best gains of your life. You'll be introduced to a

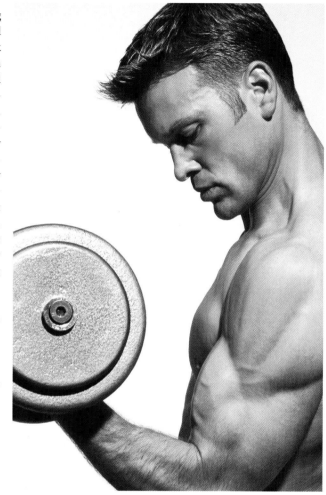

completely new way to train. Instead of doing a pre-determined number of sets, your body will determine how many you do. That allows you to work your muscles to their maximum capacity for maximum results. The end product: You'll achieve better results in less time than ever before.

You might as well get started. Chapters 1 and 2 explain the principles behind the diet and exercise program, which will help you understand the reasons that we have you eat and train the way we do. The workouts begin in Chapter 3. We've also included an "Instant Answers" chapter after each phase of the diet and workout plan. If you have any questions about a workout or diet, simply flip to the "Instant Answers" section for that phase and you'll probably find what you're looking for.

There are many different ways to achieve the same goal. But we think this is the fastest, safest and most effective method. After you've tried it, we're pretty sure you'll agree with us.

Adam Campbell
Fitness Editor, Men's Fitness®

PART I

THE
BASICS

CHAPTER 1 ▶

The Principles of Effective Training

GUYS ARE DRAWN TO WEIGHTS. It's almost an instinctive attraction, like ballparks in the summer and overpriced, state-of-the-art sound systems. Trouble is that innate desire to lift doesn't translate into iron-pumping expertise. In fact, most guys are going about it all wrong. That's because the foundation of their training philosophy is based on one highly flawed principle: More is better.

It's a widely held belief in other endeavors. Of course, you only have to apply that reasoning to fast-food consumption to know that it's not a universal truth. Just like supersize combo meals, the routines that most guys do are simply too excessive. And that limits their ability to maximize muscle growth.

You might find that hard to believe, since guys everywhere are building muscle even as you read this. But remember, we didn't say that they aren't building muscle; we said they aren't *maximizing* it. The fact is that most guys who work out follow a similar routine. It's typically something along the lines of three sets of six to eight exercises – and sometimes more – for each body part. Now consider this: That's the same type of plan that professional bodybuilders have promoted since the '80s. So the obvious question is: Are you a professional bodybuilder? Probably not. (And if you've ever seen them in the off-season, you wouldn't want to be.)

The point is: You need a workout that's designed for you. The ideal training plan is one that requires you to do the least amount of work in order to achieve the best gains. That's logical, right? It ensures that you don't sell your muscles short, overwork them or waste your time.

We'll be honest; we don't know you. Maybe you've never lifted weights before. Maybe you've been lifting for years. A conventional bodybuilding plan might work well for you and it might not. Either way, it's not likely to be optimal. That's why we're going to show you the secret to discovering the perfect plan for building *your* perfect body.

The information that follows will help you understand the training program that we provide later in the book. No matter what your experience level is, you'll be able to personalize the program for your needs. More importantly, you'll be able to use the training principles presented here to help you create your workouts long after you've finished this book. After all, if you want to keep achieving the best results, your workouts have to grow with your muscles.

THINK OBJECTIVELY

One of the biggest mistakes you can make in the gym is trying to accomplish too many goals at once. That's because the shortest path to fast gains is having one primary objective. In fact, from this point on, consider that your No. 1 rule to lift by. It should encompass every aspect of your workout program, right down to the individual exercises you perform. Think of it in terms of a math class. Typically, you're exposed to one concept at a time. Once you've grasped that concept, you're exposed to another. This allows each concept to build on the previous so that by the end of the semester, your body of knowledge has grown significantly. Problems arise when you're exposed to several concepts at once or additional concepts before you're ready. That typically makes it hard to understand any of them. It's called TMI – too much information – and it's one of the reasons that it's harder to learn from one teacher than it is from another. Some demand a rate of progression that is just too fast.

Your body is the same way. It strives to be efficient. Each time you sufficiently challenge your body physically, it makes adaptations so that the task is easier to perform the next time you do it. For instance, if you haven't exercised in a long time and try to run a mile, it'll feel extremely difficult. You may not even be able to finish it without walking. However, if you repeat that mile every other day, it'll get easier and easier. That's because your body is adapting to the training stimulus of your 1-mile run. By intelligently applying the right training stimulus for your body, you can dictate the adaptations that occur. That's the function of a good workout plan. However, trying to force your body to adapt to too many training stimuli at once is counterproductive.

For example, the most common exercise objective for most guys is to gain muscle and lose fat. The problem is that those are actually two different objectives. It's very difficult to add a significant amount of muscle while los-

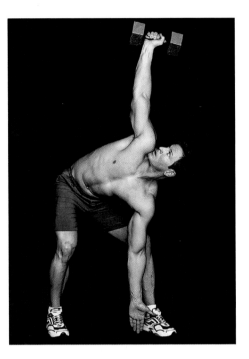

ing a significant amount of fat. The reason: To build muscle, you need an excess of calories; to lose fat, you need a shortage of calories. So the two are diametrically opposed – at least nutritionally (this is covered to a greater extent in Chapter 2). That's not to say it's impossible to lose fat while building muscle, but it's a much slower process than trying to do each separately. Most of the time, you'll be disappointed with your results. That's why we present two different plans in this book: one for adding muscle size, the other for losing fat. Trying to accomplish one of these goals at a time will result in more muscle and less fat than if you had tried to achieve them simultaneously.

Each individual workout will have a primary objective as well. That means that every repetition of every set of every exercise will be designed to accomplish that goal. This will allow you to make the fastest adaptations possible. And that means you'll sculpt a leaner, more muscular body in less time than ever before.

Bottom line: Pick one main goal and direct all of your training efforts toward achieving it.

USE THE RIGHT FORMULA

It probably doesn't surprise you when we say building muscle requires work. But by work, we're actually referring to mechanical work. That probably sounds familiar if you've ever taken a physics class. (Don't worry; it will be more interesting this time.) Work measures the transfer of energy from one object to another – for instance, your muscles to a barbell – and it can be calculated by multiplying "force" times "distance." In the world of weightlifting, force is the weight of the bar and distance is the total number of times you lift it. For example, if you perform three sets of 10 repetitions with 100 pounds, the total volume of work you performed is 3,000. The idea is to increase that number every workout by lifting heavier weights, increasing your repetitions or doing more sets. This allows you to challenge your muscles a little more with each workout, which stimulates them to grow. This is known as progressive overload.

However, you probably realize your muscles are affected differently by doing three sets of three repetitions with a heavy weight and two sets of 20 repetitions with a light weight, even if the light workout results in a greater volume of work. That's because the heavy workout is more intense. Intensity refers to the percentage of weight that you're lifting compared to the most that you can lift one time, commonly known as your one-repetition maximum. (Or simply, your "max.") The heavier the weight, the higher your intensity. This means you'll work a greater number of muscle fibers with each repetition than you would at a lower intensity. You'll also put a greater amount of tension on your muscles. This combination increases the rate of protein breakdown – a symptom of muscle damage – after your workout and leads to greater growth if you allow ample time for the muscle fibers to repair. The downside: The higher the intensity, the lower the volume of work that your muscles will be able to perform, limiting growth.

Now let's re-examine the heavy and light workout. Even though three sets of three repetitions with a heavy weight results in a high rate of protein breakdown, the volume is too low to produce significant growth. And although two sets of 20 repetitions with a light weight yields adequate volume, the intensity is too low to induce a high rate of protein breakdown. So the trick to maximizing muscle growth is to perform the ideal volume at the ideal intensity for your body. How do you know what that is? Keep reading.

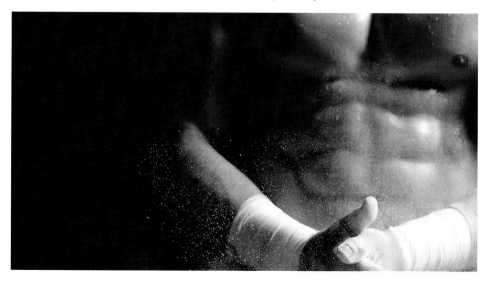

PRACTICE CLEAR COMMUNICATION

You already know that to make your muscles grow, you have to use them. But your muscles are made up of thousands of fibers, many of which rarely get used by the average guy. So to maximize growth, you have to increase your ability to use as many muscle fibers as possible. And that's dependent on how well your central nervous system – your brain and spinal cord – is able to communicate with those fibers.

Think of your central nervous system as the command center for your muscles. When you prepare to lift an object, it quickly estimates the number of muscle fibers that need to fire to complete the task. It then sends that information to those specific fibers through a nerve pathway, recruiting them for duty. This causes your muscles to contract, allowing you to generate enough force to lift the object. And this all happens in milliseconds.

The more force that's needed to lift an object, the more muscle fibers that are worked. That's why it makes sense to lift heavy weights. However, your ability to generate force is dependent on how well the nerve pathways between your central nervous system and muscles are developed for that specific movement. For example, if a guy who has never lifted before performs a bench press, he'll probably feel awkward and weak as he does the exercise. That's because the communication between his central nervous system and muscles is poor. So even though he may be muscular, his ability to use those muscles is impaired. With training, that communication improves quickly, allowing him to simultaneously recruit a greater number of muscle fibers. This is called neuromuscular adaptation. And the end result is increased strength. It's the reason why beginners often double their strength in a very short time, even before they add a significant amount of muscle.

It's important to understand the role that your central nervous system plays because asking it to do too much at one time can just confuse it, limiting the quality of your results. Imagine trying to write a detailed e-mail while you're talking on the phone. One typically distracts your attention from the other, reducing your ability to communicate effectively in either. The same thing happens when you provide too many training stimuli to your central nervous system. You won't achieve the degree of

> You need to consider the effect your training stimulus has on your central nervous system at **every level** of your workout

neuromuscular adaptation that you need to improve maximally.

The fact is that you need to consider the effect your training stimulus has on your central nervous system at every level of your workout – including the number of repetitions and sets you do, as well as the types of exercises you perform. The central nervous system is probably the most overlooked factor in creating an effective workout program. But we're going to show you how to account for it in all aspects of your training.

PLAY THE HIGH-LOW GAME

If you took a poll, you'd find that most guys perform their exercises in the same repetition range from week to week, month to month and year to year. It's usually because that's what someone told them to do when they first started lifting and they've stuck with it or because they tried a variety of repetition ranges and found one that they feel works best. For almost everyone, that number falls somewhere between five and 12 repetitions. Some guys swear by doing six repetitions per exercise, other guys think 10 is the best. The truth is that they're both right – and wrong. That's because sets that involve five to 12 repetitions provide the greatest balance of intensity and volume to maximize muscle growth. However, for the best gains, you have to expose your muscles to the full spectrum of repetitions, not just one end or the other. Here's why.

Repetitions in the lower range – five to seven – emphasize the growth of the contractile units of a muscle fiber. This also contributes to strength development, since it allows the muscle fiber to generate greater force. So if you aren't getting stronger, you aren't maximizing your ability to add muscle size.

Higher repetitions – in the range of 10 to 12 – increase the number of energy-producing structures in the muscle fiber. This in turn increases the fluid volume in the muscle fiber, which increases its size. However, this type of muscle growth doesn't contribute to strength. You might recognize this as a typical repetition range for bodybuilders, which is why they have bigger muscles, but may not be as strong as powerlifters, who use heavier weights and fewer repetitions.

A repetition range in the middle of these – six to eight – influences both types of growth, which is why you often read about lifting medium-heavy weights to maximize muscle growth.

Generally, you don't want to train in these repetition ranges in the same session. Doing so forces your body to make too many different adaptations, which reduces the effectiveness of your training. You should instead perform these repetition ranges in different sessions of the same training program. For example, in your first upper-body workout of the week you might use the lower-repetition range; in the second upper-body workout you might use the higher-repetition range. This gives your muscles time to adapt equally to each range.

CUSTOMIZE YOUR SETS

Just as guys favor specific rep ranges, they also stick with the same number of sets for long periods of time. The default is usually three sets per exercise. The reason? It just seems to work. But it could work a lot better.

There's no real logic behind performing three sets. Guys will typically use this scheme

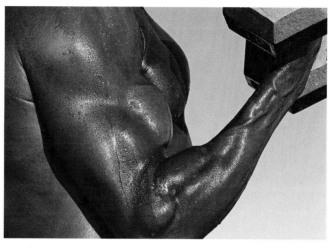

with several exercises per body part and call it a workout. But as they move from exercise to exercise, they end up using weights that don't adequately challenge the muscle fibers, diluting the training stimulus. The other problem is that it's a cookie-cutter approach. While some guys only require a couple of sets for maximum gains, others might need six or seven.

We have a simple solution: Let your body decide. How? Simply do as many sets as it takes to achieve "technical failure." You might be familiar with the term failure as it pertains to lifting. It's generally understood to be the point at which you can't perform one more repetition, usually accompanied by a bulging forehead vein and a loud-mouthed spotter yelling, "It's all you, man, it's all you." (For the record, it's rarely "all you.") As popular as this technique is, it's actually counterproductive to your muscle gains. That's because it requires you to engage different muscles than those you're targeting to lift the weight and takes a toll on your central nervous system. That not only slows recovery, it requires your muscles and central nervous system to adapt to stimuli above and beyond your objective – both of which limit muscle growth.

Technical failure, on the other hand, is the point at which there is a break in your form. This is a bit subjective, but with a little practice you can easily learn to identify it. Any time there is a decrease in your bar speed or a change in body posture, consider it a break in form. For example, if you're performing the bench press and your bar speed slows when you hit your "sticking" point, you've just achieved technical failure. And whether you've done two sets or six sets, you're finished with that exercise. Likewise, if you catch yourself leaning backward or forward to complete an arm curl, you're done. Simply monitor your own form, rep by rep, and you'll know when technical failure occurs.

MASTER WEIGHT MANAGEMENT

Using the appropriate weight is a critical factor in maximizing your gains. You want to challenge your muscles without over-challenging them. You basically want them to work as hard as they need to in order to achieve the results you desire. This is pretty tricky for most guys

> Any time there is a decrease in your bar speed **or a change in body posture**, consider it a break in form

because there's always the problem of ego. You've heard the phrase "Check your ego at the door," but have you ever put it to use? Probably not. Guys tend to overestimate themselves in almost every capacity (ask any ex-girlfriend) and lifting is no exception. So even if you have the best intentions, you're still likely to use a weight that's heavier than you need. That means you'll achieve technical failure faster, which will limit the work that you're able to do.

The weight you use should allow you to perform each prescribed repetition of your first set with perfect form. In other words, you shouldn't reach technical failure. If that's not possible, you've started off too heavy. For instance, at one point in the size and strength phase of our workout plan, you'll be required to perform sets of seven repetitions with a weight that's equal to your seven-repetition maximum. However, that doesn't mean the heaviest weight you can lift seven times by any means possible; it means the heaviest weight you can lift seven times while maintaining perfect form. That's a key difference that most guys ignore. It's OK if you achieve technical failure in your second set – that will vary by person – but you should by no means achieve it in your first set. If you do, you're defeating the purpose of performing your seven-repetition maximum. (If we want you to perform your six-repetition maximum instead, we'll tell you.)

It's simple: To achieve the specific adaptation that each workout is striving for, you have to do the workout the way that it's prescribed. Otherwise, you're reducing its effectiveness.

WORK ABROAD

We've already discussed the importance of total work for building muscle. And you'll find that as you perform the workouts and become better trained, you'll gradually be able to increase the amount of work you can do. For instance, you'll discover that it takes more repetitions each workout to reach technical failure. That's because you're adapting to the training stimulus and improving your work capacity.

Work capacity refers to the total amount of work you can perform in a single workout. It's different for every person. That's why some guys can do a greater number of sets than others. Consider work capacity the foundation of your training pyramid: the wider the base, the higher your peak – the potential for muscle size and strength gains – can be.

Thankfully, there's a way to increase your work capacity beyond what you accomplish in your weight-training program, especially if you're new to lifting. It's called energy system training. Its function – for our purposes – is to increase your level of fitness specifically for lifting weights.

We stress specificity because the beauty of energy system training is that it can be customized to improve work capacity for any type of activity – for instance, running or cycling or sports, like basketball and soccer.

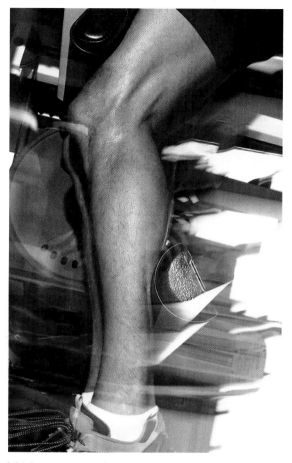

It used to be that improving fitness levels meant training your aerobic energy system. (That's why coaches made football players jog laps to get in shape.) Unfortunately, they were misguided. The adaptations your body makes to a training stimulus is specific to the type of training you do. So if you run laps for 30 minutes, you'll improve your ability to run laps for 30 minutes. In other words, aerobic activities – like long, slow distance running – improve aerobic performance. Football is anaerobic, meaning it requires energy for short bursts of high-intensity exercise. Think about it: The average play lasts about six seconds and it typically involves an all-out effort. So running short sprints would be a specific form of training that would improve fitness levels for football.

The same is true for weightlifting, since it's also an anaerobic activity. Typically, a set lasts anywhere from 10 seconds to one minute and is challenging for the entire duration. So if you want to improve your work capacity outside the weight room, you'll want to train using activities that match the typical duration and intensity of the sets that you perform in your strength workout. Most of the time that means performing intervals by alternating high-intensity sprints with adequate rest periods.

Intervals not only increase your work capacity, they're also beneficial for fat loss, especially compared to aerobic exercise. In a study at Laval University in Quebec, researchers found that guys who performed high-intensity intervals lost three times more fat than guys who did low- to moderate-intensity aerobic training, even though the aerobic guys exercised longer and burned more than twice as many calories. So energy system training not only helps you do more work, it's ideal for using as part of fat-loss plan.

KEEP IT SIMPLE

Even though much of our program uses techniques that you may not have tried before, you won't have any trouble recognizing the exercises. We stick with the basics for one simple reason: Basic exercises allow you to use the heaviest weight possible. That means you'll be able to apply the maximum amount of tension to your muscles for any prescribed repetition range. Remember: more tension, more muscle.

You may have noticed that over the last few years, Swiss balls have become extremely popular. In fact, they have an almost cult-like following. The idea is that by performing exercises such as the chest press, shoulder press and arm curl while lying or sitting on the Swiss ball, you put your body in an unstable environment, forcing your central nervous system to work harder, while training the muscles that stabilize your body – your abs, back and hips – at the same time. The problem is that this requires you to use lighter weights to compensate for your body's instability, which reduces the tension on your muscles. For instance, you can lift heavier weights while doing chest presses lying on a bench as opposed to a Swiss ball. So if your goal is to increase the muscle size of your chest, you reduce the effectiveness of the exercise by performing it on a Swiss ball.

In addition, while doing exercises on a Swiss ball is taxing to your central nervous system, it's not necessarily beneficial. Because Swiss balls require your body to recruit additional muscle fibers to maintain stability, your central nervous system has to communicate with more parts of the body simultaneously. This takes away from the development of the nerve pathways between your central nervous system and the muscles that you're trying to build. The end result is that your central nervous system works hard, but the work isn't focused where it needs to be to reach your goal.

That said, Swiss balls can be useful for increasing the range of motion of some exercises – such as abdominal crunches – as well as improving body weight exercises. But you don't need them to get big arms or a big chest.

DO YOUR PREP WORK

The warm-up is typically the most ignored part of a training program. And that's certainly understandable, since it's time-consuming and doesn't seem to yield benefits that you can see in the mirror. But the right warm-up will actually improve your performance, helping you to achieve your primary objective faster.

There are usually two types of warm-ups: general and specific. A general warm-up should warm your muscles, increasing blood flow and improving your joint flexibility and range of motion. Most guys use aerobic exercise machines, such as the treadmill, stationary

> The right warm-up will actually **improve your performance**, helping you to achieve your primary objective faster

bike and stair climber, to accomplish this. Unfortunately, that type of warm-up isn't just boring, it's extremely unproductive. It only increases the temperature of a few muscles and doesn't have a significant impact on flexibility. It also entirely ignores your upper body. A better method is to use a series of compound exercises performed with a light weight and low repetitions. This increases the temperature of *all* the muscles that you'll use in your workout, without resulting in fatigue. It also doubles as a dynamic flexibility workout, meaning it improves your ability to perform movements through a greater range of motion. That's important because it ensures that you'll work your muscles through their complete functional range, allowing you to stimulate a greater number of muscle fibers.

A specific warm-up is simply lighter weight sets of the exercise that you're about to perform. The goal is to engage your central nervous system and remind it of the movement pattern – for instance, a bench press – that you'll be doing. This increases your body's ability to recruit more muscle fibers simultaneously, allowing you to lift heavier weights. Think of a specific warm-up as a primer for your central nervous system.

More guys do this type of warm-up as opposed to a general one. The problem is that they usually botch it up by doing too many repetitions. For instance, a lot of guys use a pyramid routine, starting with higher repetitions and lighter weights and gradually progressing to lower repetitions and heavier weights. This is counterproductive because you waste valuable energy by performing too many repetitions – typically 10 to 15 per set – in the first two or three sets. A ramping method is a better approach. You keep the repetitions low the entire time and do a minimal number of sets. This prevents you from using up too much energy, while still preparing your central nervous system for the heavy weights to come. Remember, you warmed your muscles in the general warm-up, so that's not your objective with the specific warm-up. Here's an example of an effective ramp-up warm-up. The percentages shown relate to the amount of weight that you'll use in first work set.

Set 1: Five repetitions with 55 to 60 percent.

Set 2: Three repetitions with 75 to 80 percent.

Set 3: One repetition with 90 to 95 percent.

Following this scheme, if you'll be using 200 pounds in your first set of the bench press, you might use 110 pounds in the first warm-up set, 160 pounds in the second warm-up set and 185 pounds in the third warm-up set. The percentages aren't critical, but you can use them as a guideline. If you're lifting extremely heavy weights – 400 pounds on the squat, for instance – you might try performing two or three additional warm-up sets with smaller increases in weight. The key is to keep your repetitions to a minimum.

Once you've performed a specific workout for a muscle group (for instance, chest), you don't need to warm up again if you perform another exercise that works that same muscle group.

EMBRACE DOWNTIME

Your muscles grow when they're resting, not working. That's when the adaptations from your training stimulus take place. If you work a muscle group too often, you won't allow it to adapt completely, which defeats the purpose of training it in the first place. The result is less

> **FACT ►**
>
> **Recovery time is extremely variable and highly subjective: What might be ample rest for one guy might not be enough for another, even if they're doing identical workouts**

than ideal gains in muscle and strength size. Rest days aren't a luxury, they're a requirement. In general, you shouldn't train more than four days a week or you won't allow yourself enough recovery time.

Your central nervous system needs time to recover from a hard workout, too. This is a highly overlooked factor in most training plans. Follow this rule of thumb: The higher the intensity of your workout, the greater the demand on your central nervous system. So as you lift closer to your one-repetition maximum, you should perform less total volume. That is, the heavier you lift, the fewer total sets you do and vice versa. (Our method of performing sets until technical failure automatically adjusts volume for increases in intensity.) Otherwise, your central nervous system will be taxed too hard and your ability to recover between workouts will be compromised.

All that said, recovery time is extremely variable and highly subjective. What might be ample rest for one guy might not be enough for another, even if they're doing identical workouts. Besides adjusting the volume of work for intensity, as well as limiting the total number of days you train, you need to monitor your results and body for markers of over-reaching, a state of physiological fatigue. A decrease in performance from workout to workout is the first indication of physiological fatigue. Keep a training log to track your progress. Think of each workout as a reassessment. If the amount you can lift, or the number of repetitions or sets you can do, decreases from one workout to the next, you need to increase the number of rest days between your workouts. If the total volume of work you can do increases from workout to workout, keep the amount of rest the same.

Other signs of over-reaching include decreased appetite, an increase or decrease in your blood pressure, an increased eye-blink rate (usually someone will mention it to you) and a lower sex drive (someone might mention this to you, too). You can also monitor this by checking your pulse right after you wake in the morning. It should only vary by three to five beats per minute from day to day; any more raises the concern of over-reaching.

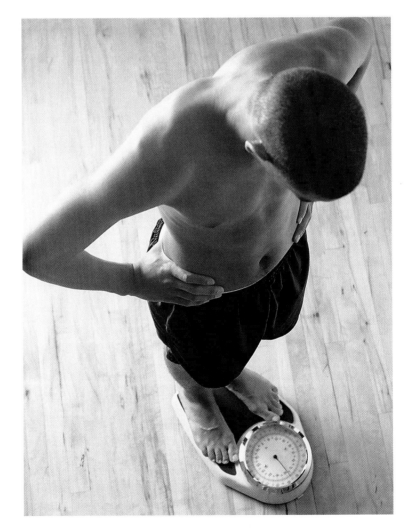

CHAPTER 2 ▶

Nutrition: Your Recipe For Success

ABS ARE MADE IN THE KITCHEN."

We certainly didn't coin this phrase, but it perfectly sums up the importance of smart eating. No matter what your goal is, the fastest path to dramatic results is through your stomach. Think of your ideal body as a recipe: Your diet provides the right ingredients in the right amounts to achieve the results you want. If you give your body too much of the wrong types of foods, or too little of the right types of foods, you'll spoil the recipe.

That's not to downplay the importance of working your muscles. Exercise is a requirement. But even a turbo-blender can't turn a doughnut into a protein shake. If you want a chiseled body, your nutrition plan has to be as sound as your workout plan. Your first step is understanding the ingredients.

THE MAJOR PLAYERS

From your body's perspective, you eat to provide it with essential nutrients, as well as energy, measured in calories. Your body acquires energy from four sources. The first three – carbohydrates, protein and fat – are known as macronutrients. The fourth is alcohol. Knowing the amount of energy that each of these yields, and understanding the way each affects your metabolism, will help you increase the rate at which your body builds muscle or loses fat. Let's start with the basics.

CARBOHYDRATE

Carbohydrates contain about four calories per gram and are classified as either simple or complex. Conventional nutrition advice is to avoid simple carbohydrates – especially for fat loss – and eat plenty of complex carbohydrates. Unfortunately, it's a flawed recommendation. To fully understand why, you first need a complete explanation of each.

Simple carbohydrates. These are the "sugars" of the carbohydrate family. They're divided into two categories: monosaccharides, or "single" sugars, and disaccharides, or "double" sugars.

There are three main types of monosaccharides: glucose, your body's primary source of energy;

fructose, a sugar that occurs naturally in fruits and honey, and galactose, which is rarely present in foods by itself. Each of these monosaccharides has the same number and type of atoms, but they're arranged differently, giving them distinct chemical structures.

Disaccharides are composed of two monosaccharides. All of these pairs include glucose. For instance, sucrose – commonly known as table sugar – is a combination of glucose and fructose; and lactose, or milk sugar, is a combination of glucose and galactose.

Complex carbohydrates. These are polysaccharides, meaning they're composed of more than two single sugars. Think of them as chains of monosaccharides held together by chemical bonds. The three major polysaccharides that you eat are glycogen, starch and fiber. Glycogen is the stored form of glucose in animals and is only available in meat. It's typically not a significant source of carbohydrates or calories. Starch is the stored form of glucose in plants. There's an abundance of starch in vegetables, such as potatoes, corn and legumes, as well as in bread, rice, oats and any other form of grain. Fiber is the structural material of plants in the stems, leaves, roots and skins. It's found in vegetables, fruit, grains and legumes.

How It Works. Glucose is the chemical form of carbohydrate that your body uses for energy. Unless you're consuming a very low carbohydrate diet, it's your body's primary energy source. (Your body is burning fat and protein at the same time, but the greatest percentage of energy is coming from carbohydrates.) A very low carbohydrate intake forces your body to conserve glucose and burn fat preferentially.

Glucose is already in the form that your body needs, so it's quickly digested and absorbed into your bloodstream. (The word "sugar" in "blood sugar" refers to glucose.) Because it's absorbed rapidly, glucose consumption rapidly raises your blood-sugar level. This stimulates the release of insulin, a hormone that keeps your blood-sugar level normal.

Unfortunately, elevated insulin levels signal your body to stop burning fat. This allows your body to increase the rate at which it burns glucose for energy in order to lower your blood-sugar levels back to normal as fast as possible. At the right times and with the right combination of nutrients – as you'll see later in this chapter – insulin spikes can be beneficial for building muscle. However, if you're trying to lose fat or minimize the fat you gain, frequently eating foods that are composed of glucose will have a detrimental effect on achieving your goals.

Disaccharides always contain glucose, so they fall into the category of foods that rapidly increase your blood-sugar and insulin levels. Interestingly, so do many complex carbohydrates. Since starch is stored glucose, your body can quickly digest and absorb it. However, that depends on an important factor. Namely, fiber.

Fiber is considered a "non-available" carbohydrate because human digestive enzymes can't break down the chemical bonds that hold its chains of monosaccharides together. So in general, fiber doesn't yield any direct energy. That's why high-fiber, low-starch vegetables such as broccoli are low in calories. Fiber also has a beneficial effect on the digestion and absorption of starch. It slows the breakdown of starch into glucose and delays its absorption into your bloodstream, decreasing the insulin response associated with a high-starch food. The problem is that processing removes fiber from many foods. White and whole-grain bread, for example, are both made from wheat flour. But the flour is highly refined when it's used for white bread, increasing the speed of digestion and absorption, and resulting in a greater release of insulin.

Luckily, there's a simple way to choose your foods without having to know their starch and fiber content. It's called the glycemic index. The glycemic index of a food describes its effect on blood sugar. Understanding the impact of glucose on your blood-sugar levels will help you make wise food choices. The higher the glycemic index, the faster the food raises your blood sugar. Choose carbohydrates that are high in fiber and have a low glycemic index (known as low-glycemic foods) to keep insulin levels low and allow your body to burn fat at a higher rate. (For the glycemic index of common foods, go to www.glycemicindex.com.

We should also say a few words about fructose. When you eat fructose, it's digested and absorbed into your bloodstream and then sent to the liver to be converted into glucose. Although it doesn't cause a rapid rise in blood sugar, or a significant spike in insulin, fructose is preferentially converted into fat in the liver.

Don't bag fruit forever. Small amounts of fructose – like those found in oranges, apples and pears – are unlikely to impair your ability to lose fat. In fact, when researchers at Vanderbilt University added a small amount of fructose to a drink containing high amounts of glucose, they found that the glycemic response was 19 percent lower than it was with a glucose-only drink. In addition, fresh fruit is high in fiber and contains valuable antioxidants that lower your risk for disease. The problem arises when fructose is consumed in large quantities. High-fructose corn syrup, a sugar substitute made from fructose (55 percent) and glucose (45 percent), is the major culprit.

During the past 30 years, high-fructose corn syrup has replaced sucrose as the primary sweetener in processed foods. It's used everywhere: soda, juice, candy, cereal and even condiments. Between 1971 and 1997, the same time frame in which obesity rates skyrocketed, consumption of this sweetener rose 351 percent. Avoid these products as much as possible by reading food labels. High-fructose corn syrup is often the first ingredient listed.

PROTEIN

For years, only bodybuilders appreciated the nutritional benefits of protein. But research shows that the nutrient is just as important for fat loss as it is for muscle growth. Like carbohydrates, protein contains about four calories per gram. It's composed of different amino acids that are linked together by chemical bonds. There are 20 types of amino acids, 11 of which are nonessential, meaning your body can make them. The other nine are essential and must be supplied to your body by your diet in order for you to survive.

ESSENTIAL AMINO ACIDS

Histidine
Isoleucine
Leucine
Lysine
Methionine
Phenylalanine
Threonine
Tryptophan
Valine

NON-ESSENTIAL AMINO ACIDS

Alanine
Arginine
Asparagine
Aspartic acid
Cysteine
Glutamic acid
Glutamine
Glycine
Proline
Serine
Tyrosine

Unlike simple and complex carbohydrates, there aren't different categories of protein. However, the quality of protein varies. Proteins that contain all nine essential amino acids are high quality and the best for building muscle. In general, almost any food that comes from an animal – beef, chicken, fish, eggs and dairy for example – contains high-quality protein. Supplements such as whey and casein protein – both milk-derived – are also high quality.

Except for soy, most plant proteins are incomplete, meaning they lack at least one of the essential amino acids. Therefore, in order to acquire all of the essential amino acids to create a complete protein, vegetables have to be eaten in combination. This is why it's hard for vegetarians, especially vegans, to consume the ideal amount of high-quality protein for adding muscle.

How It Works. Your body uses protein for a variety of functions, including tissue repair, enzyme and hormone formation, and nutrient transportation. Proteins can also be converted to glucose – a process called gluconeogenesis – and used as energy. And, of course, there's a connection between protein and muscle.

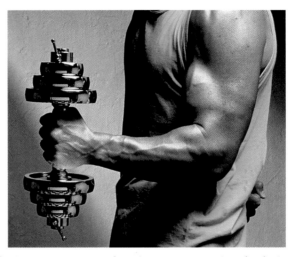

Muscles are basically stored protein. When you eat protein, it's digested and broken down into amino acids. The amino acids are absorbed and released into the bloodstream, then delivered to the sites in the body where new proteins are needed. This is where amino acids are assembled into new proteins, a process known as protein synthesis.

Your body's protein stores are in a continuous state of turnover. That is, as new proteins are built, old ones are broken down and used for one of their many functions. If protein synthesis occurs at the same rate as protein breakdown, you are in protein balance. (In other words, it's a wash.) For muscle growth to occur, you have to create a positive protein balance, which ensures that your body has a surplus of raw materials to increase its protein stores, or muscle.

If you undereat, your body converts a greater amount of protein to glucose for energy, leaving you in protein balance, or worse, a negative protein balance. This is why crash-dieters lose muscle and why it's difficult to simultaneously gain muscle and lose fat. Creating a positive protein balance requires you to not only consume an ample amount of high-quality protein, but an ample amount of total calories as well.

FAT

Fat contains about nine calories per gram, more than twice that of carbohydrates and protein. That's one of the main reasons why nutritionists recommend that you eat a low-fat diet. (You can eat a greater amount of food if it contains less fat.) The problem is that people took this message to heart, eating carbohydrates to their stomach's content. The USDA confirms this,

reporting that since 1971, Americans' calorie intake has risen by more than 500 calories a day, enough to gain a pound a week.

Fat is probably the most complicated and misunderstood of the three macronutrients. Ninety-five percent of the fat that you eat in food, as well as the fat that your body stores, is known as a triglyceride. The other 5 percent is composed of phospholipids – important parts of cell membranes – and sterols, the kind of fat that includes cholesterol and hormones, such as testosterone. However, for the purpose of understanding the function of fat, we'll just examine triglycerides.

A triglyceride is composed of three fatty acids that are attached to a glycerol molecule. (Without getting into complicated biochemistry, just know that glycerol serves as the "backbone" for the fatty acids.) If amino acids are the building blocks of protein, then fatty acids are the building blocks of a triglyceride.

Fatty acids vary in size and can be either saturated or unsaturated, which is a chemist's way of describing their structure. You're probably familiar with the terms saturated fat, monounsaturated fat and polyunsaturated fat. These are all triglycerides with a different structure of chemical bonds. Saturated fats are typically solid at room temperature, while unsaturated fats are liquid. All fatty acids are basically chains of four to 24 carbon atoms. They might be referred to as short-chain (less than six carbons), medium-chain (six to 10 carbons) or long-chain (12 to 24 carbons) fatty acids. This also allows them to be specifically identified, such as an 18-carbon saturated fatty acid.

Monounsaturated and polyunsaturated fats are generally considered healthy fats, although that can be dependent on the chain length of the fatty acids. Saturated fats are typically considered unhealthy. However, it's interesting to note that 18-carbon stearic acid, a saturated fat commonly found in chocolate and beef, appears to be harmless and is an excellent energy source, while 12-, 14- and 16-carbon saturated fatty acids appear to be the most dangerous since they have the greatest cholesterol-raising effect. This isn't necessarily important to know for the purposes of building muscle or losing fat, but it does illustrate the bigger picture of how different kinds of fat can affect your body.

Just like there are essential amino acids, there are also essential fats. These are the fats that your body needs to live and they must come from your diet. There are two: linoleic acid, known as an omega-6 fatty acid, and linolenic acid, known as an omega-3 fatty acid. Both are polyunsaturated fats. Most Americans get plenty of omega-6 fatty acids, since they're abundant in meats and vegetable oil. omega-3 fatty acids are found in fatty fish – such as salmon, tuna and mackerel – as well as walnuts, flaxseed and canola oil.

How It Works. Your body digests fat into fatty acids, glycerol (the backbone) and monoglycerides. (Monoglycerides are "smaller" versions of triglycerides, since they only have one fatty acid attached to their glycerol backbone.) Short-chain and medium-chain fatty acids are absorbed directly into your bloodstream, where they become free-fatty acids and are available for the body to use as energy. They're the preferred energy source of your heart and muscles while you're at rest.

Long-chain fatty acids and monoglycerides are built back into triglycerides, but aren't immediately absorbed into the blood because long-chain fatty acids are insoluble in water, which is the foundation of blood. Instead they're packed into delivery vessels called lipoproteins and transported to various sites throughout the body for use as energy, insulation and the construction of cell structures. Contrary to popular opinion, fat isn't immediately stored as fat, since it has many functions to perform within the body. However, if you consume more energy than your body needs, it does store fat for later use. The amount it stores, however, depends on how it's combined with the other macronutrients, as well as your body's overall metabolic environment. It's important to note, though, that fat doesn't induce an insulin response. Eating fat by itself doesn't signal your body to store fat. In fact, it keeps your body burning fat, since it signals that fat is readily available in your diet and doesn't need to be stored.

ALCOHOL

Alcohol contains about seven calories per gram. Your body absorbs alcohol, or more accurately ethyl alcohol – the kind in alcoholic beverages – very quickly and it classifies it as a toxin. So it metabolizes alcohol before the macronutrients (carbohydrates, fat and protein) in order to dispose of it as fast as possible. This means that your body's ability to burn fat is impaired when alcohol is present, since alcohol takes precedence. A drink a day probably won't significantly affect your results, especially if the rest of your diet is in line. However, if you binge drink or make heavy drinking a regular habit, you'll drastically reduce the effectiveness of your diet and exercise plan.

PLAYING THE PERCENTAGES

Now that you understand the main ingredients – carbohydrate, fat, protein and alcohol – you need to do some simple math. Add up the number of grams of each macronutrient that you eat and multiply those values by their respective energy content to determine how many total calories you're taking in at any given time. So if you eat a meal that contains 30 grams of protein, 40 grams of carbohydrate and 14 grams of fat, you'd perform the following calculation:

30 grams of protein x 4 calories per gram	= 120 calories
40 grams of carbohydrate x 4 calories per gram	= 160 calories
14 grams of fat x 9 calories per gram	= 126 calories
Total calories = 406	

This allows you to monitor your total intake of calories. (For a database of the macronutrient and calorie content of common foods, go to www.fitday.com.) It also allows you to control the percentage of calories that you consume from each macronutrient. Divide the calories from each macronutrient by the total number of calories consumed. In the above example, this would be:

Protein: 120 calories/406 total calories = 30 percent of total calories

Carbohydrate: 160 calories/406 calories = 39 percent of total calories

Fat: 126 calories /406 calories = 31 percent of total calories

In each phase of our diet plan, we'll recommend the percentage of calories that should come from each macronutrient, allowing you to get the right quantities of nutrients for each phase's objective.

RESULTS BY THE NUMBERS

You've heard it before: If you eat more calories than you burn, you'll gain weight; if you eat fewer calories than you burn, you'll lose weight. This is a bit of an oversimplification, but it's a good rule of thumb. You need to know how many calories you can eat without gaining or losing any weight. This will allow you to

target your energy intake – or total daily calories – to achieve your goals as fast as possible.

Even while you're at rest, your body is constantly burning calories to keep your heart beating, kidneys functioning and lungs breathing. The energy required to perform these activities is called your resting metabolic rate. This varies by person and depends primarily on body size. You also burn more calories through basic daily activities such as walking from the parking lot to your car, brushing your teeth and even digesting your food. In other words, virtually any activity your body is involved in requires energy, which burns calories. Of course, you also have to account for the calories you burn while you're working out.

There are many different formulas for predicting your daily caloric expenditure. For this book, we'll use the one in the box on the next page:

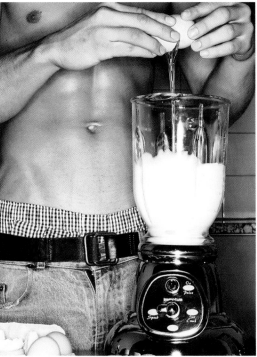

DAILY CALORIC EXPENDITURE FORMULA		
A. Your weight in pounds		=
B. Multiply A by 11 to get your resting metabolic rate	**A** x 11	=
C. Multiply B by 1.6 to estimate your caloric expenditure through basic daily activities	**B** x 1.6	=
D. Strength training: Multiply the number of minutes you lift weight per week by 5:	min. x 5	=
E. Aerobic and sprint training: Multiply the number of minutes per week that you run, cycle or play sports by 8	min. x 8 =	
F. Add line D and line E, and divide by 7	**(D + E)**/7 =	
G. Add line C and line F to get your daily calorie needs:	**C + F**	=
		Total

The final result (line G) is an estimate of the total number of daily calories you require to maintain your weight. (We'll call this "maintenance.") If you increase your total calorie intake above this number, you'll gain weight. By decreasing your total calorie intake, you'll lose weight. That's why our program includes two distinct plans: the Maximum Muscle Phase and the Full-Scale Fat-Loss Phase. The key is to avoid extremes. For instance, one pound is equal to approximately 3,500 calories. Ideally, to lose a pound of fat a week, you'd reduce your calorie intake by 500 calories a day below maintenance. However, there's a limit to the effectiveness of reducing calories. If you reduce them too much, your metabolism will slow to conserve energy, reducing your ability to burn fat. In addition, the more calories you cut, the greater your risk of losing muscle along with the fat. Low-calorie diets also reduce testosterone levels, the key hormone for muscle-building. So put a cap on calorie reduction at 1,000 calories a day, assuming that keeps you in the neighborhood of a 2,000-calorie-a-day diet. (For instance, if your maintenance is 2,700, you'll just cut out 700 calories a day.) Following this plan (as you will in our Full-Scale Fat-Loss Phase), you can expect to lose about two pounds of fat per week.

Calculating your calorie needs for building muscle is a little more difficult. Your goal is to gain as much muscle as possible without adding a significant amount of fat. For this, you'll shoot to increase your maintenance by 500 calories a day. Whether or not this is enough depends on your individual metabolism and how closely the formula approximated your actual caloric needs.

Try the diet plan for a week. The day you begin, weigh yourself in the morning, after you've gone to the restroom, but before you eat breakfast. The following week, weigh yourself again, following the same procedure. If you haven't gained one pound, increase your calorie intake by 250 calories a day. Continue this process each week until you're gaining a pound a week. (Don't worry; we'll cover this again in the Maximum Muscle Phase.) Your body can only build muscle so fast, so increasing your caloric intake too much will just result in an increase in fat on top of your muscle gains. In other words, you'll gain more weight, but you won't add a great deal more of muscle.

WINNING COMBINATIONS

You've just taken a crash course in nutrition. It's important to understand the details, but you can also boil it all down to some very general guidelines. If you stick with these concepts, while monitoring your total calories according to your goals, you'll have great success in this program.

THE GOLDEN RULES OF CLEAN EATING

1. Eat protein at every meal. Eating protein all day long ensures that there is plenty available when your body needs it to make muscle.

Regardless of whether you're trying to gain muscle or lose fat, consume about one gram of protein per pound of body weight. (If you weigh 180 pounds, you'll eat 180 grams of protein.) A study in the *Journal of Applied Physiology* found this was the maximum amount that your body can use in a day. We generally recommend that you eat five to six meals a day, equally dividing your protein intake between each meal, especially if your goal is to gain muscle. In the example used earlier, you'd eat six meals each day, consuming 30 grams of protein at each meal.

Protein impacts fat loss as well. The more protein you eat, the more calories you can eat. That's because the thermic effect of protein is 25 to 30 percent, compared to 6 to 8 percent for carbohydrates and about 2 percent for fat. So by simply replacing some carbohydrates with protein, you can help speed weight loss.

2. Avoid eating high-glycemic foods with fat.
Remember what happens when you eat carbohydrates that quickly raise your blood sugar? Your body releases insulin to help lower it back to normal, which simultaneously shuts down its ability to burn fat. It also signals your body to start storing fat. So if you combine high-glycemic carbohydrates with a hefty serving of fat, you're providing the raw materials to increase your fat stores. The more fat you eat, the more fat that becomes readily available to be packed away in the fat cells between your skin and your abs. However, if you avoid eating these two types of food simultaneously, the effect isn't as severe. Insulin will still inhibit your body's ability to burn fat, but you won't be aiding the enemy by providing it with extra soldiers.

Keep in mind that you want to eat plenty of fat. So eating fat with high-fiber foods that have a low-glycemic index is not only acceptable, it's recommended.

3. Eat before and after your workout.
Research shows that eating protein right before and immediately following your workout increases the rate of protein synthesis and decreases the rate of protein breakdown. So either way, you build muscle faster. But we recommend that you hedge your bet and eat both times, ensuring maximum muscle growth.

The diet plans in this book instruct you to vary the quantity and type of calories that you consume depending on whether your primary objective is to gain muscle or lose fat. Either way, we recommend that you consume high-glycemic carbohydrates – along with protein – after your workout. That's probably surprising

> **THE GOLDEN RULES OF CLEAN EATING ▶**
> **1.** Eat protein at every meal
> **2.** Avoid eating high-glycemic foods with fat
> **3.** Eat before and after your workout

to you considering that everything else you've read about high-glycemic carbohydrates, particularly their effect on insulin levels. However, insulin comes in handy after your workout. Just as it inhibits the use of fat for energy, it inhibits the use of protein for energy. So it's very effective at reducing protein breakdown when consumed with plenty of amino acids (read: high-quality protein). And that speeds muscle growth.

In addition, consuming high-glycemic carbohydrates immediately after your workout affects your metabolism differently than at other times of the day. That's because the carbohydrates are preferentially used to replenish the glucose stores, or glycogen, in your muscles.

Fair warning: Neglecting to eat before or after your workout will reduce your ability to maximize your gains in muscle, as well as the rate at which you lose fat.

CHAPTER 3 ▶

Results Start Here

YOU'RE ABOUT TO EMBARK ON A COMPLETE TRAINING REGIMEN designed to pack on muscle and melt fat, sculpting your body faster and more effectively than ever before. Since you'll achieve the best results by focusing on one goal at a time, there are four separate phases in this program. Here's a snapshot of each:

*The Preparation Phase: Work Capacity (3 weeks)

Note: This phase is optional. To determine if you should start with this phase, use the "Work Capacity Assessment" on page 30. If you don't qualify to start with the Maximum Muscle phase, you may be tempted to jump into it anyway. Don't. You'll achieve much better results by following our recommendations precisely.

These workouts in the preparation phase will improve your work capacity for the Maximum Muscle phase by increasing your level of fitness specifically for weight training.

Phase 1: Maximum Muscle (6 weeks)

The workouts in this phase will increase your muscle size and strength. Any fat that you gain in this phase will be burned off in the Full-Scale Fat-Loss phase. Overall, this workout and diet combination will allow you to add maximum muscle with minimal fat.

Phase 2: Full-Scale Fat-Loss (6 weeks)

These workouts are geared to accelerate your rate of fat loss, while maintaining your hard-earned gains from the Maximum Muscle phase.

The Bonus Phase: Chest and Arm Specialization (4 weeks)

This is the trophy-muscle workout. Designed to emphasize muscle gains in your chest and arms, it's the perfect way to finish off our plan.

BEFORE YOU BEGIN

Each workout in this book recommends one of the two following warm-up sessions. Each will warm up your muscles, precondition your connective tissues and prime your central nervous system to lift heavy weights. These objectives will take your body from its normal resting state to a level of optimized functional potential that will allow you to execute each exercise with maximum effort and minimum risk of injury. Use the following warm-ups as recommended in each workout.

WARM-UP 1

Perform the warm-up exercises as a circuit, doing one exercise after the next without resting. After you've completed the circuit, briefly catch your breath then repeat until you've completed the number of circuits prescribed in each workout. Do five repetitions of each exercise with an unloaded barbell (45 pounds). After you've completed all of your circuits, proceed to the first exercise of your workout.

1. Overhead Squat
2. Squat
3. Good Morning
4. Lunge
5. Romanian Deadlift
6. Bent-over Row

WARM-UP No. 2

Perform the warm-up exercises as a circuit, doing one exercise after the next without resting. After you've completed the circuit, briefly catch your breath then repeat until you've completed the number of circuits prescribed in each workout. Do each exercise for 30 seconds, using only your body weight. Once you've performed the exercise for the prescribed duration, move on to the next. After you've completed all of your circuits, proceed to the first exercise of your workout.

1. Jumping Jack
2. Split Jack
3. Prisoner Squat
4. Alternating Lunge
5. Mountain Climber

THE PREPARATION PHASE: WORK CAPACITY

This three-week cycle includes two parts: weight training and energy system training. Follow the directions below for each. Regardless of your initial fitness level, you should be able to complete three full circuits without extended rest periods (no more than two minutes) by the end of the three-week cycle. If you can't, repeat the three-week cycle before moving on to the Maximum Muscle Workout. (For diet, follow the Maximum Muscle Diet starting on page 97. It will give you a head start for the Maximum Muscle phase.)

THE WEIGHT WORKOUT

Warm-up: Do three to five circuits of Warm-up No. 1 before you do Workout A, and three to five circuits of Warm-up No. 2 before you do Workout B.

Frequency: Alternate between Weight Workout A and Weight Workout B three days a week for three weeks, resting one day between each workout. For example, in Week 1 you'll perform

WORK CAPACITY ASSESSMENT

If any of the statements below apply to you, follow the Three-Week Work Capacity Program prior to initiating the Maximum Muscle Workout.

1. You've never performed any form of strength training.

2. You haven't exercised at all in the past two weeks.

3. You haven't done any weight training in the past two weeks after a period of consistent weight training lasting at least three months.

4. You've just completed a training cycle specifically designed to raise your one-repetition maximum in a major lift such as the squat, the bench press or the deadlift.

5. You've recently recovered from an injury that required you to take time off from exercise or significantly modify your exercise program.

6. Your strength-training experience has not included the use of free weights.

Weight Workout A on Monday and Friday, and Weight Workout B on Wednesday. In Week 2, you'll perform Weight Workout B on Monday and Friday, and Weight Workout A on Wednesday.

Exercise Order: Perform the exercises as a modified circuit by doing one exercise after the next (in the order shown), but resting in between each. So you'll do one set of the first exercise, rest, one set of the second exercise, rest and so on until you've completed one set of each movement. Your rest periods between exercises and sets should not exceed two minutes. Rest only until your breathing approaches normal.

Repetitions and Weights: For each exercise (except where noted), use the heaviest weight that allows you to complete all of the prescribed number of repetitions of the first set without achieving technical failure. So if you're supposed to do 20 repetitions, use a weight that's equal to your 20-repetition maximum. This will take a little experimentation, but you should have it down by the second time you do the workout. You'll need to increase the weight that you're using for each exercise every week, since the repetitions decrease.

Week 1: Do 20 repetitions of each exercise.
Week 2: Do 15 repetitions of each exercise.
Week 3: Do 12 repetitions of each exercise.

ENERGY SYSTEM TRAINING

Perform these workouts on the days between your weight workouts. Perform Energy System Training (EST) A on the day following Weight Workout A. Do EST B on the day following Weight Workout B. So in Week 1, you'll perform EST Workout A on Tuesday and Saturday,

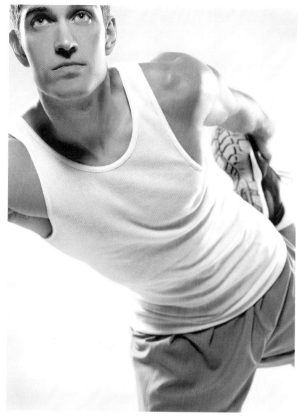

and EST Workout B on Thursday. In Week 2, you'll perform EST B on Tuesday and Saturday, and EST A on Thursday.

WORKOUT A

Week 1: Run at a pace that's about 65 percent of your full effort for 20 minutes.
Week 2: Run at a pace that's about 70 percent of your full effort for 20 minutes.
Week 3: Run at a pace that's about 75 percent of your full effort for 20 minutes.

WORKOUT B

Week 1: Run at a pace that's about 70 percent of your full effort for 20 minutes.
Week 2: Run at a pace that's about 75 percent of your full effort for 20 minutes.
Week 3: Run at a pace that's about 80 percent of your full effort for 20 minutes.

AT A GLANCE: THE PREPARATION PHASE

	Monday	Tuesday	Wednesday	Thursday	Friday	Saturday	Sunday
Week 1	WW A	EST A	WW B	EST B	WW A	EST A	rest
Week 2	WW B	EST B	WW A	EST A	WW B	EST B	rest
Week 3	WW A	EST A	WW B	EST B	WW A	EST A	rest

AT A GLANCE: WORKOUT A

EXERCISE	INTENSITY	SETS	REPS
Warmup #1	Bar	3-5	5
1. Drop Squat			
Week 1	20RM	2-3	20
Week 2	15RM	2-3	15
Week 3	12RM	2-3	12
2. Underhand-grip Dumbbell Row			
Week 1	20RM	2-3	20
Week 2	15RM	2-3	15
Week 3	12RM	2-3	12
3. Reverse Hyperextension			
Week 1	20RM	2-3	20
Week 2	15RM	2-3	15
Week 3	12RM	2-3	12
4. Elbows-in Elevated Pushup			
Week 1	20RM	2-3	20
Week 2	15RM	2-3	15
Week 3	12RM	2-3	12
5. Side Bridge			
Week 1	Body	2-3	10
Week 2	Body	2-3	10
Week 3	Body	2-3	10
6. Side Lateral Raise and Rotation			
Week 1	20RM	2-3	20
Week 2	15RM	2-3	15
Week 3	12RM	2-3	12

AT A GLANCE: WORKOUT B

EXERCISE	INTENSITY	SETS	REPS
Warmup #1	Bar	3-5	5
1. Multidirectional Lunge			
Week 1	20RM	2-3	20
Week 2	15RM	2-3	15
Week 3	12RM	2-3	12
2. Underhand-grip Dumbbell Row			
Week 1	20RM	2-3	20
Week 2	15RM	2-3	15
Week 3	12RM	2-3	12
3. Single-leg Bridge			
Week 1	Body	2-3	10
Week 2	Body	2-3	10
Week 3	Body	2-3	10
4. Serratus Dip			
Week 1	20RM	2-3	20
Week 2	15RM	2-3	15
Week 3	12RM	2-3	12
5. Plank			
Week 1	Body	2-3	10
Week 2	Body	2-3	10
Week 3	Body	2-3	10
6. Hanging Scapular Retraction			
Week 1	Body	2-3	10
Week 2	Body	2-3	10
Week 3	Body	2-3	10

Overhead Squat

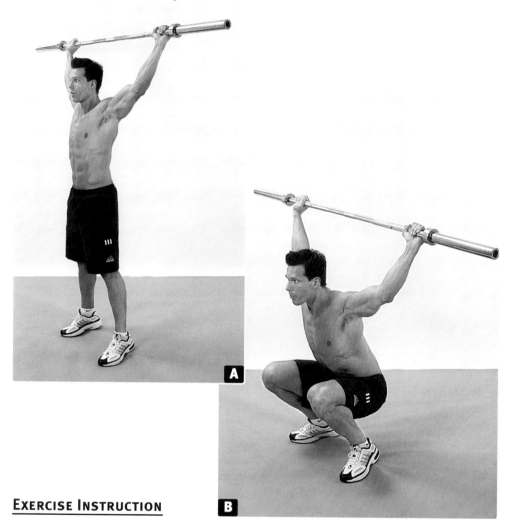

EXERCISE INSTRUCTION

(A) Hold a barbell with an overhand grip that's twice the width of your shoulders and press it up so that your arms are fully extended above your head. The bar should be directly over your shoulders. Set your feet shoulder-width apart, keeping your back naturally arched, and squeeze your shoulder blades together.

(B) Slowly lower your body as far as possible, keeping your back in its natural alignment, and the barbell directly above your shoulders at all times. Pause, then return to the starting position.

WARM-UP 1

Squat

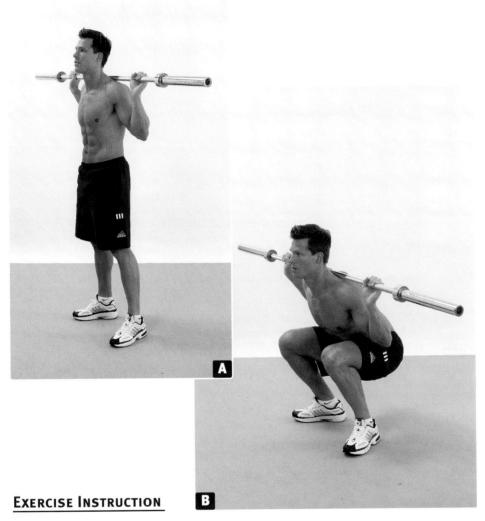

A

B

EXERCISE INSTRUCTION

(A) Hold a bar across your upper back with an overhand grip, feet shoulder-width apart and your shoulders pulled back.

(B) Slowly lower your body as far as possible – or until your thighs are at least parallel to the floor – keeping your back naturally arched and your lower legs nearly perpendicular to the floor.

Pause, then return to the starting position.

Good Morning

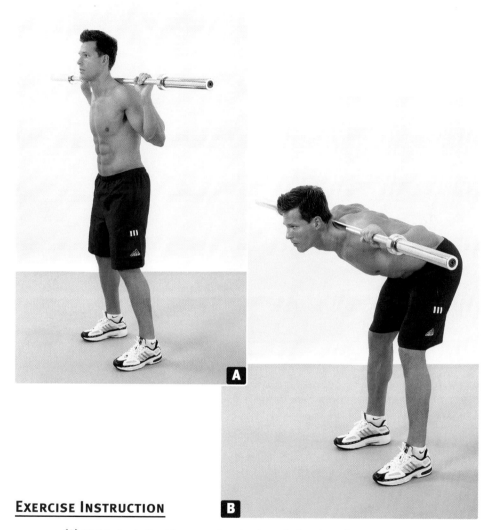

EXERCISE INSTRUCTION

(**A**) Hold a barbell with an overhand grip and place it so that it rests comfortably across your upper back. Bend your knees slightly.

(**B**) Slowly bend forward at the hips, maintaining the arch in your lower back as you lower your chest as far as you can or until your upper body is parallel to the floor. Keep your head up and maintain the slight bend in your knees throughout the lift.

Pause and then lift your upper body back to the starting position.

WARM-UP 1

Barbell Lunge

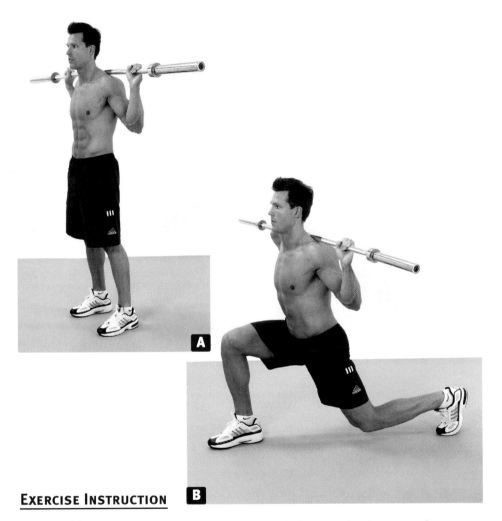

EXERCISE INSTRUCTION

(A) Grab a barbell with an overhand grip and place it so that it rests comfortably across you upper back. Stand with your feet hip-width apart.

(B) Step forward with your left leg and lower your body until your front knee is bent 90 degrees and your rear knee nearly touches the floor. Your front lower leg should be perpendicular to the floor and your torso should remain upright.

Push yourself back up to the starting position as quickly as you can, and repeat with your right leg. That's one repetition.

Romanian Deadlift

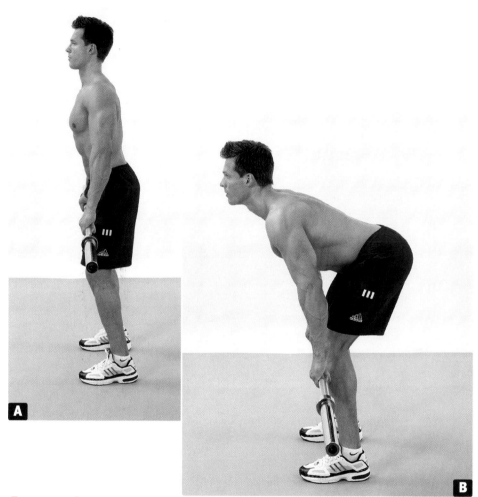

EXERCISE INSTRUCTION

(A) Grasp a bar with an overhand grip that's just beyond shoulder-width and hold it at arm's length, resting it on the front of your thighs. Your feet are shoulder-width apart and your knees are slightly bent.

(B) Slowly bend at the hips, keeping your lower back naturally arched – as you lower it against your body until it's just below your knees. Maintain the same angle of your knees throughout the lift.

Lift your torso back to the starting position, keeping the bar as close to your body as possible.

WARM-UP 1

Bent-over Row

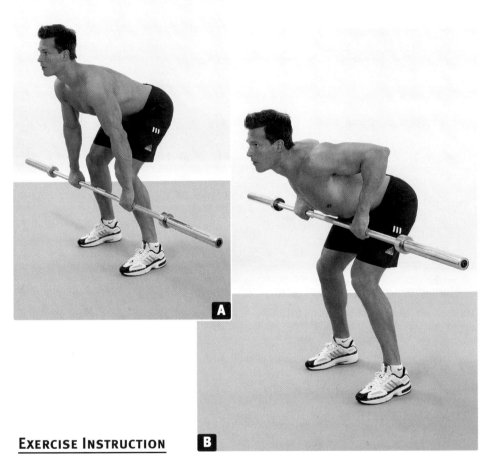

EXERCISE INSTRUCTION

(A) Grab a barbell with an overhand grip that's just beyond shoulder width, and hold it at arm's length. Stand with your feet shoulder-width apart and knees slightly bent. Bend at the hips, keeping your lower back naturally arched, and lower your torso until it's almost parallel to the floor. Let the bar hang straight down from your shoulders.

(B) Pull the bar up to your torso, pause, then slowly lower it.

Jumping Jack

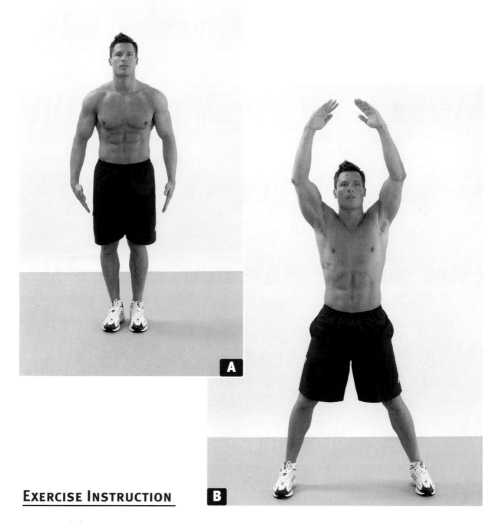

EXERCISE INSTRUCTION

(A) Stand with your feet together and your hands at your sides.

Simultaneously raise your arms above your head and jump up just enough to spread your feet a few inches.

(B) Without pausing, quickly reverse the movement and repeat as many times as you can.

WARM-UP 2

Split Jack

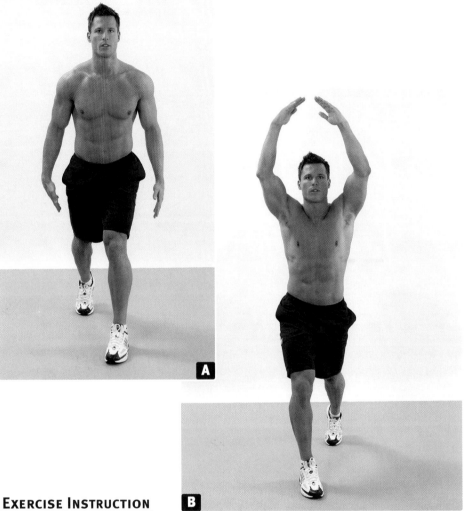

EXERCISE INSTRUCTION

(A) Stand with your feet together and your hands at your sides.

Simultaneously raise your arms above your head and jump back with one foot and forward with the other.

(B) Without pausing, quickly switch legs back and forth as you continue to raise and lower you arms. Repeat as many times as you can in the allotted time period.

Prisoner Squat

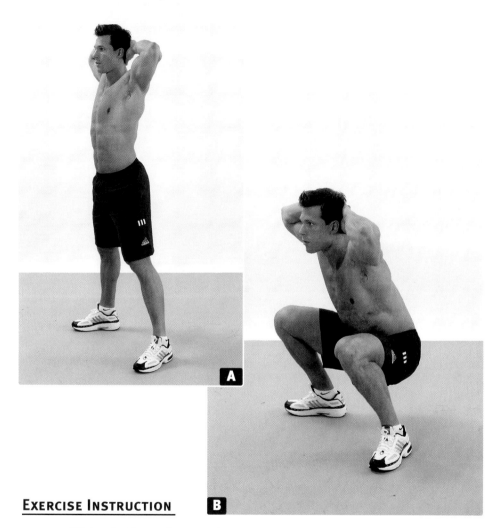

EXERCISE INSTRUCTION

(A) Stand with your feet apart about twice the width of your shoulders and your hands behind your head.

(B) Lower your body as far as possible – or until your thighs are at least parallel to the floor – keeping your back naturally arched and your lower legs nearly perpendicular to the floor.

Pause, then return to the starting position.

WARM-UP 2

Alternating Lunge

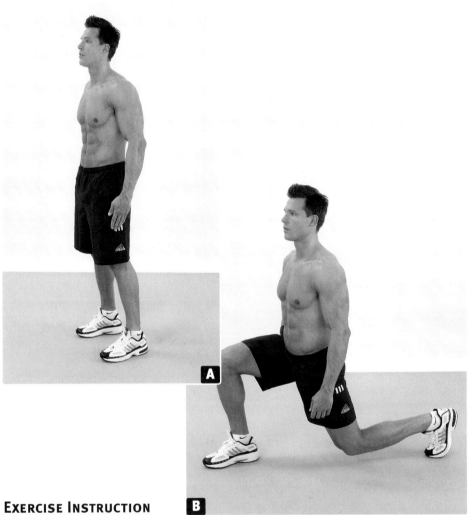

EXERCISE INSTRUCTION

(A) Stand with your feet hip-width apart and your hands at your sides.

(B) Step forward with your left leg and lower your body until your front knee is bent 90 degrees and your rear knee nearly touches the floor. Your front lower leg should be perpendicular to the floor and your torso should remain upright.

Push yourself back up to the starting position as quickly as you can and repeat with your right leg. That's one repetition.

Mountain Climber

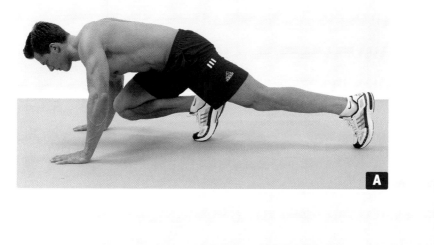

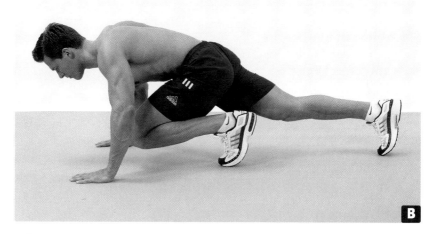

EXERCISE INSTRUCTION

(A) Kneel on all fours, your hands in line with and slightly wider than your shoulders. Straighten your left leg so that only the balls of your feet are touching the floor. Lift your right knee toward your chest so that only the balls of your feet are touching the floor. (You should look like a sprinter that's in the starting blocks.)

(B) Quickly switch leg position as many times as you can for the allotted time period.

WORKOUT A

Drop Squat

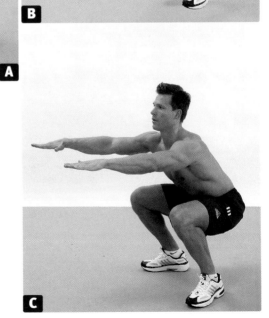

EXERCISE INSTRUCTION

(A) Stand with your feet shoulder-width apart, your arms completely straight in front of your body so that they're parallel to the floor.

(B) Simultaneously jump up so that your feet leave the floor as you lower your body until your thighs are parallel to the floor.

(C) Return to the starting position and repeat.

Underhand-Grip Dumbbell Row

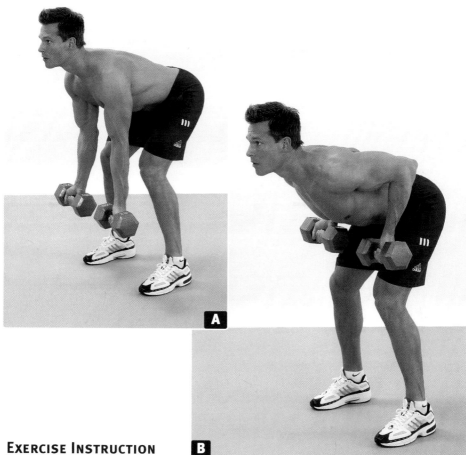

EXERCISE INSTRUCTION

(A) Grasp a pair of dumbbells with an underhand grip. Stand with your feet shoulder-width apart and knees slightly bent. Keeping your back naturally arched, bend at the hips and lower your torso until it's almost parallel to the floor. Let the dumbbells hang straight down from your shoulders, palms facing out.

(B) Pull the dumbbells up to your torso, pause, then slowly lower it.

WORKOUT A

Reverse Hyperextension

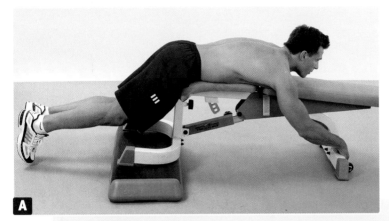

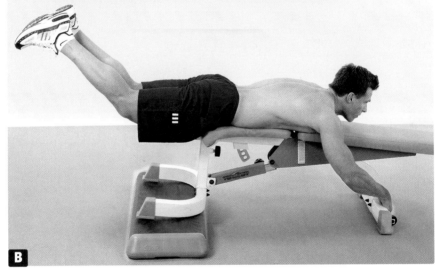

EXERCISE INSTRUCTION

(A) Lie on a bench so that your arms are at the end of the bench where your feet normally go. Place your body so that your abdomen is resting on the bench and your hips are completely off of it. Keep your legs together and straight, with your body forming a straight line. (This works best on a higher surface. You can place one end of the bench on an aerobic step if needed.) Slowly lower your legs to the floor.

(B) Pause, then lift your hips and thighs until they're in line with your torso.

Elbows-in Elevated Push-up

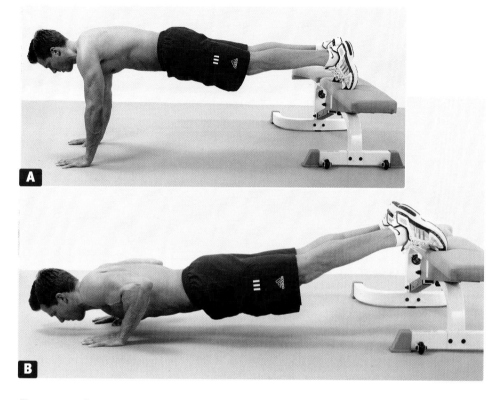

EXERCISE INSTRUCTION

(A) Get into push-up position – your hands set slightly wider than and in line with your shoulders – with your arms straight. Place your feet on a bench or other elevated, sturdy surface.

(B) Without allowing your hips to sag, lower your body until your chest nearly touches the floor, keeping your elbows as close to your torso as possible.

Pause, then push yourself back up to the starting position.

WORKOUT A

Side Bridge

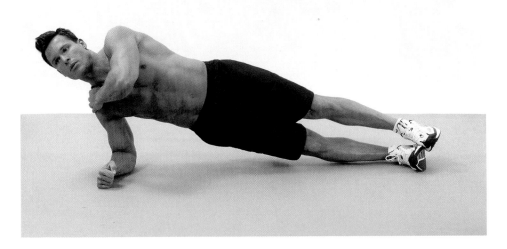

EXERCISE INSTRUCTION

Lie on your right side with your knees straight. Prop your upper body up on your right elbow and forearm, which should be directly below your right shoulder. Place your left hand on your right shoulder and raise your hips until your body forms a straight line from your ankles to your shoulders.

Contract and brace your abdominals. Hold this position for five seconds, breathing steadily. That's one repetition.

Each week, add an additional five seconds to the duration of the repetition, so that you're holding 10 seconds the second week and 15 seconds the third week.

Side Lateral Raise and Rotation

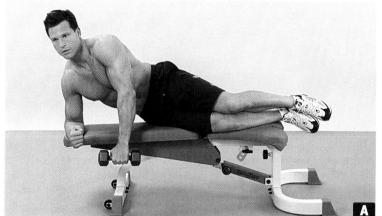

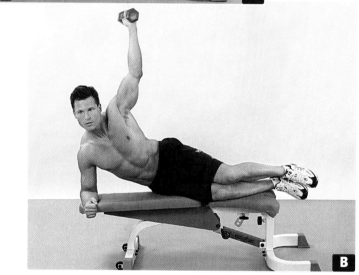

EXERCISE INSTRUCTION

(A) Hold a dumbbell in your right hand and lie on your left side on a flat bench. Prop yourself up with your left elbow. Let your right arm hang straight down from your body so that it's perpendicular to the floor, your palm turned toward you, elbow slightly bent.

(B) Without changing the bend in your elbow, raise your arm above your shoulder, while rotating it so that your palm is facing your head.

Reverse the movement and repeat.

WORKOUT B

Barbell Lunge

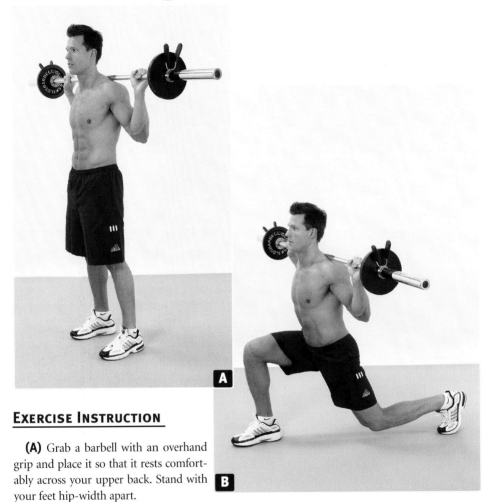

EXERCISE INSTRUCTION

(A) Grab a barbell with an overhand grip and place it so that it rests comfortably across your upper back. Stand with your feet hip-width apart.

(B) Step forward with your left leg and lower your body until your front knee is bent 90 degrees and your rear knee nearly touches the floor. Your front lower leg should be perpendicular to the floor and your torso should remain upright.

Push yourself back up to the starting position as quickly as you can, and repeat with your right leg. That's one repetition.

Single-Leg Bridge

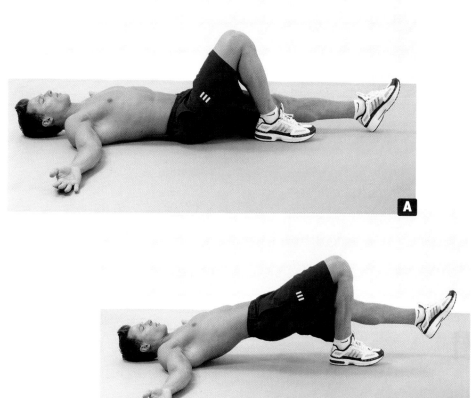

EXERCISE INSTRUCTION

   (A) Lie on your back on the floor with your left knee bent and your right leg straight.

   (B) Raise your hips so your body forms a straight line from your shoulders to your left knee.

   Lower hips to return to the start position.

   After you've completed all of the prescribed repetitions, repeat with your right knee bent and your left leg straight.

WORKOUT B

Serratus Dip

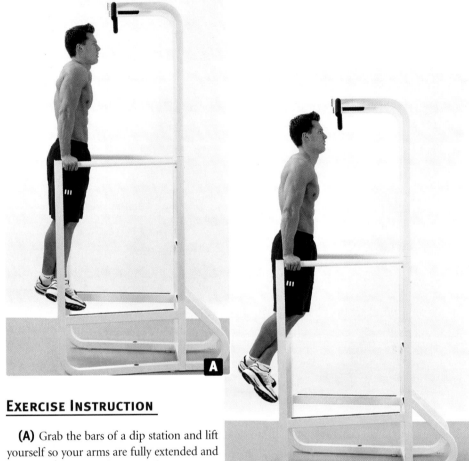

EXERCISE INSTRUCTION

(A) Grab the bars of a dip station and lift yourself so your arms are fully extended and locked. Bend your knees and cross your ankles behind you.

(B) Without changing your arm position, press your shoulders down as you lift your upper body. (In other words, "shrug" your shoulders down instead of up.)

Pause, then return to the starting position. (If this is too easy, wear a dipping belt or hold a dumbbell in the bend of your knees.)

Plank

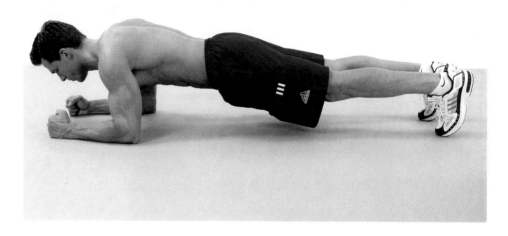

EXERCISE INSTRUCTION

Get into push-up position: Arms are straight and directly below your shoulders, legs are extended straight back behind you. Bend your elbows and rest your weight on your forearms. Your body should form a straight line from your shoulders to your ankles.

Contract and brace your abdominals. While breathing steadily, hold this position for five seconds. That's one repetition.

Each week, add an additional five seconds to the duration of the rep, so that you're holding 10 seconds the second week and 15 seconds the third week.

WORKOUT B

Hanging Scapular Retraction

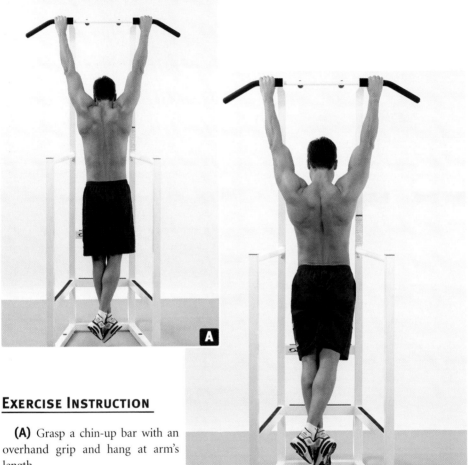

EXERCISE INSTRUCTION

(A) Grasp a chin-up bar with an overhand grip and hang at arm's length.

(B) Without moving your arms, pull your shoulder blades down and together. Hold this position for five seconds, breathing steadily. That's one repetition.

Each week, add an additional five seconds to the duration of the rep, so that you're holding 10 seconds the second week and 15 seconds the third week.

PART II

THE
MAXIMUM
MUSCLE
PHASE

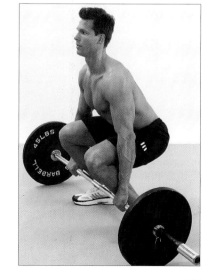

CHAPTER 4 ▶

Maximum Muscle Workout

THIS SIX-WEEK CYCLE INCLUDES TWO PARTS: weight training and energy system training. Follow the directions for each. Combine this workout plan with the Maximum Muscle Diet on page 97.

THE WEIGHT WORKOUT

STAGE 1: WEEKS 1 to 3

Warm-up: Do two to three circuits of Warm-up No. 1 before Workout A and Workout C, and two to three circuits of Warm-up No. 2 before Workout B and Workout D.

Frequency: Perform each workout once a week, doing Workout A and Workout B on consecutive days, resting a day or two, then completing Workout C and Workout D on consecutive days. For example, do Workout A on Monday, Workout B on Tuesday, Workout C on Thursday and Workout D on Friday.

Exercise Order: Perform the exercises using either straight sets or alternating sets. Straight sets will be designated simply as a number – for instance, "2" or "5." Alternating sets will be designated as a number and letter pair – for instance, "1A" and "1B." For straight sets, complete all sets of the exercise before moving on to the next. For alternating sets, perform one set of the first exercise, rest, then do one set of the second exercise and rest again, alternating back and forth until you've completed all sets of both exercises.

Rest: Between sets and exercises, rest only as long as it takes for your breathing rate to approach normal. This time period should never exceed two minutes.

Repetitions and Weights

Workout A: For each exercise, start with one set of seven repetitions using your seven-repetition maximum. (The heaviest weight you can lift seven times without achieving technical failure.) Then do as many sets as you can with that weight using the repetition scheme below. When you achieve technical failure, move on to the next exercise.

Week 1: 5 repetitions
Week 2: 6 repetitions
Week 3: 5 repetitions

Workout B: For each exercise, perform one set of 12 repetitions with your 12-repetition maximum. (The heaviest weight you can lift 12 times without achieving technical failure.) Then do as many sets as you can with that weight using the repetition scheme below. When you achieve technical failure, move on to the next exercise.

Week 1: 10 repetitions
Week 2: 11 repetitions
Week 3: 10 repetitions

Workout C: Do three sets of six repetitions of exercise 1. For all other exercises, start by performing one set of 12 repetitions with your 12-repetition maximum. (The heaviest weight you can lift 12 times without achieving technical failure.) Then do as many sets as you can with that weight using the repetition scheme below. When you achieve technical failure, move on to the next exercise.

Week 1: 10 repetitions
Week 2: 11 repetitions
Week 3: 10 repetitions

Workout D: Do three sets of six repetitions of exercise 1. Start by performing one set of seven repetitions with your seven-repetition maximum. (The heaviest weight you can lift seven times without achieving technical failure.) Then do as many sets as you can with that weight using the repetition scheme below. When you achieve technical failure, move on to the next exercise.

Week 1: 5 repetitions
Week 2: 6 repetitions
Week 3: 5 repetitions

ENERGY SYSTEM TRAINING
STAGE 1: WEEKS 1 to 3

Do Energy System Training (EST) A on the day following Weight Workout B. Do EST B on the day following Weight Workout D. (You'll perform EST A on Wednesday and EST B on Saturday.)

REST DAYS AREN'T A LUXURY ➤ They are a requirement. Your muscles **grow** when they are resting, not working. In general you shouldn't train more than **four days** a week

EST A
Week 1: Do six 15-second sprints at 100 percent of your full effort, resting for 60 seconds between each.

Week 2: Do eight 15-second sprints at 100 percent of your full effort, resting for 60 seconds between each.

Week 3: Do 10 15-second sprints at 100 percent of your full effort, resting for 60 seconds between each.

EST B
Week 1: Do five 30-second sprints at 100 percent of your full effort, resting for 120 seconds between each.

Week 2: Do six 30-second sprints at 100 percent of your full effort, resting for 120 seconds between each.

Week 3: Do seven 30-second sprints at 100 percent of your full effort, resting for 120 seconds between each.

AT A GLANCE: THE MAXIMUM MUSCLE WORKOUT (STAGE 1)							
	Monday	Tuesday	Wednesday	Thursday	Friday	Saturday	Sunday
Week 1	WW A	WW B	EST A	WW C	WW D	EST B	rest
Week 2	WW A	WW B	EST A	WW C	WW D	EST B	rest
Week 3	WW A	WW B	EST A	WW C	WW D	EST B	rest

AT A GLANCE: WORKOUT A (STAGE 1)

EXERCISE	INTENSITY	SETS	REPS
Warmup #1	Bar	2-3	5
1A. Incline Dumbbell Press			
Week 1	7RM	N	5
Week 2	7RM	N	6
Week 3	7RM	N	5
1B. Neutral-Grip Dumbbell Row			
Week 1	7RM	N	5
Week 2	7RM	N	6
Week 3	7RM	N	5
2. Scaption			
Week 1	7RM	N	5
Week 2	7RM	N	6
Week 3	7RM	N	5
3. Incline Lower Trap Raise			
Week 1	7RM	N	5
Week 2	7RM	N	6
Week 3	7RM	N	5

*N = the number of sets it takes you to reach technical failure

AT A GLANCE: WORKOUT B (STAGE 1)

EXERCISE	INTENSITY	SETS	REPS
Warmup #2	Body	2-3	5
1A. High Step-up			
Week 1	12RM	N	10
Week 2	12RM	N	11
Week 3	12RM	N	10
1B. Romanian Deadlift			
Week 1	12RM	N	10
Week 2	12RM	N	11
Week 3	12RM	N	10
2. Off-set Incline DB Curl			
Week 1	12RM	N	10
Week 2	12RM	N	11
Week 3	12RM	N	10
3. Incline Lower Trap Raise			
Week 1	12RM	N	10
Week 2	12RM	N	11
Week 3	12RM	N	10

*N = the number of sets it takes you to reach technical failure

AT A GLANCE: WORKOUT C (STAGE 1)

EXERCISE	INTENSITY	SETS	REPS
Warmup #1	Bar	2-3	5
1. Dynamic Pushup			
Week 1	Body	3	6
Week 2	Body	3	6
Week 3	Body	3	6
2A. Bench Press			
Week 1	12RM	N	10
Week 2	12RM	N	11
Week 3	12RM	N	10
2B. Chin-up			
Week 1	12RM	N	10
Week 2	12RM	N	11
Week 3	12RM	N	10
3. Combo Raise			
Week 1	12RM	N	10
Week 2	12RM	N	11
Week 3	12RM	N	10
4. Horizontal Lateral Raise			
Week 1	12RM	N	10
Week 2	12RM	N	11
Week 3	12RM	N	10

*N = the number of sets it takes you to reach technical failure

AT A GLANCE: WORKOUT D (STAGE 1)

EXERCISE	INTENSITY	SETS	REPS
Warmup #2	Body	2-3	5
1. Jump Squat			
Week 1	Bar	3	6
Week 2	Bar	3	6
Week 3	Bar	3	6
2A. Bulgarian Split Squat			
Week 1	7RM	N	5
Week 2	7RM	N	6
Week 3	7RM	N	5
2B. Good Morning			
Week 1	7RM	N	5
Week 2	7RM	N	6
Week 3	7RM	N	5
3. Lying DB Triceps Extension			
Week 1	7RM	N	5
Week 2	7RM	N	6
Week 3	7RM	N	5
4. Barbell Roll-out			
Week 1	7RM	N	5
Week 2	7RM	N	6
Week 3	7RM	N	5

*N = the number of sets it takes you to reach technical failure

Incline Dumbbell Press

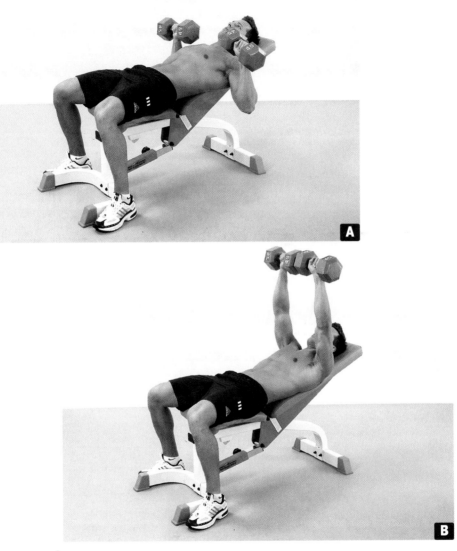

EXERCISE INSTRUCTION

(A) Holding a dumbbell in each hand, lie on your back on a bench set to a low incline (15 to 30 degrees). Bring the dumbbells to chest height, palms facing out toward your feet.

(B) Press the dumbbells up and toward each other until they almost touch and your arms are completely straight.

Slowly lower the weights to your upper chest, pause, then repeat.

Neutral-Grip Row

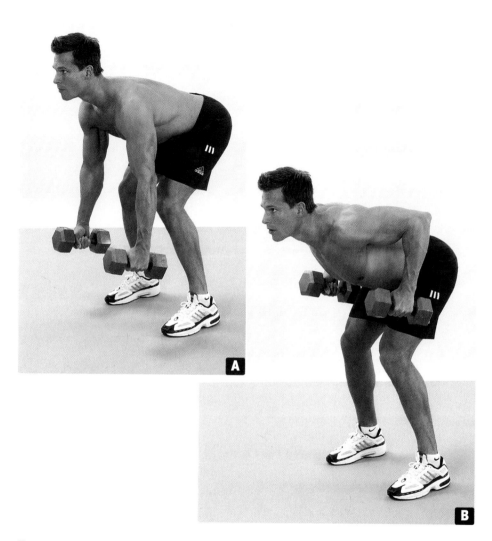

EXERCISE INSTRUCTION

(A) Stand with your feet shoulder-width apart and knees slightly bent. Grab a pair of dumbbells and hold them at arm's length at your sides. Keeping your back naturally arched, bend at the hips and lower your torso until it's almost parallel to the floor. Let the dumbbells hang straight down from your shoulders, your palms facing each other.

(B) Pull the weights up to the sides of your torso, pause, then slowly lower them.

WORKOUT A

Scaption

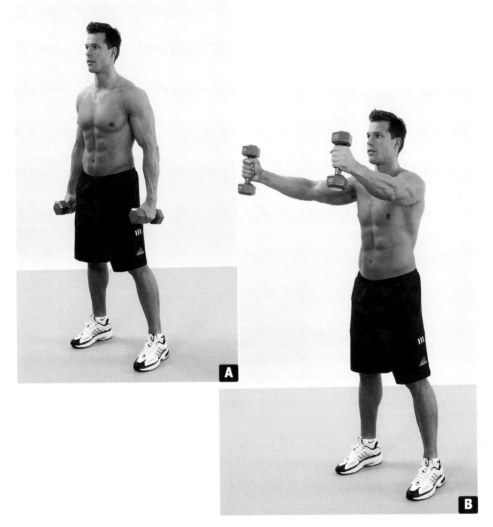

EXERCISE INSTRUCTION

(A) Stand with your feet shoulder-width apart, holding a dumbbell in each hand. Let the dumbbells hang at arm's length next to your sides, your palms facing each other and your elbows slightly bent.

(B) Without changing the bend in your elbows, raise your arms at a 30-degree angle to your body (so that they form a "Y") until they're at shoulder level.

Pause then slowly lower the weights to the starting position.

Incline Lower Trap Raise

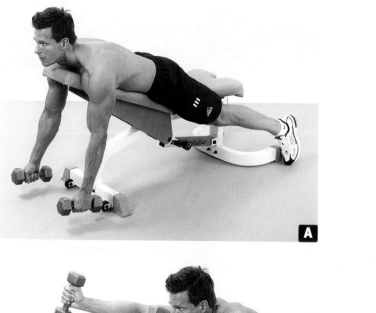

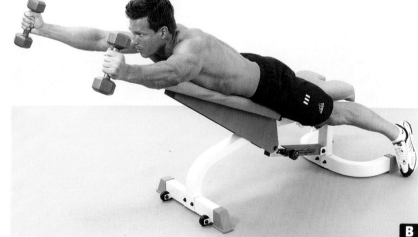

EXERCISE INSTRUCTION

(**A**) Set an incline bench to a 30-degree angle. Holding a dumbbell in each hand, lie with your chest against the pad. Let your arms hang straight down from your shoulders and turn your palms so they're facing each other. Keep your elbows slightly bent.

(**B**) Without changing the bend in your elbows, raise your arms at a 30-degree angle to your body (so that they form a "Y") until they're in line with your torso.

Pause and then slowly lower the weights to the starting position.

WORKOUT B

High Step-up

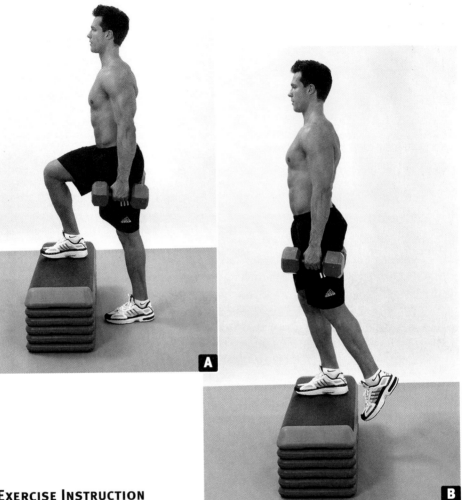

EXERCISE INSTRUCTION

(A) Holding a dumbbell in each hand, allow your arms to hang at your sides. Stand in front of a bench or step and place your right foot firmly on the bench. The step should be high enough so that your knee is bent 90 degrees.

(B) Press your right heel into the step and push your body up until your right leg is straight and you're standing on one leg on the bench, keeping your left foot elevated.

Lower your body until your left foot touches the floor. That's one repetition.

Once you've completed all of the repetitions with your right leg, repeat the exercise with your left leg.

Romanian Deadlift

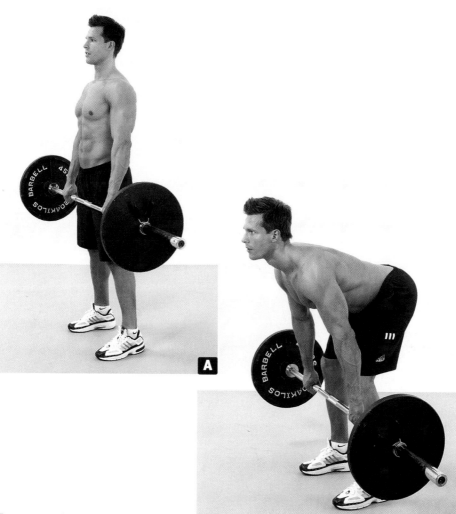

EXERCISE INSTRUCTION

(A) Hold a bar with an overhand grip that's just beyond shoulder width. Let the bar hang at arm's length in front of your thighs. Your feet are shoulder-width apart and your knees are slightly bent.

(B) Slowly bend at the hips, keeping your lower back naturally arched, as you lower the bar just below your knees. Maintain the same angle in your knees throughout the lift.

Lift your torso back to the starting position, keeping the bar as close to your body as possible.

WORKOUT B

Offset Incline Dumbbell Curl

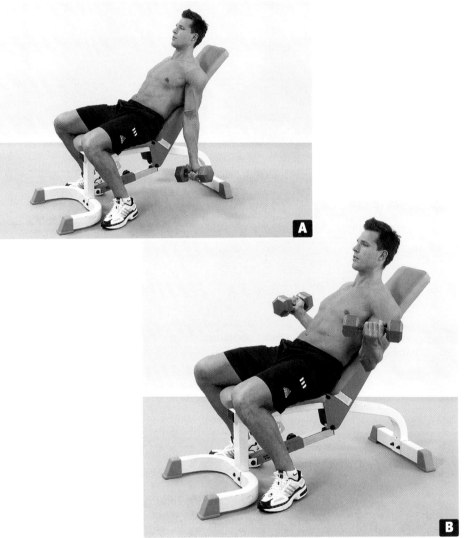

EXERCISE INSTRUCTION

(A) Set an incline bench to a 45-degree angle and hold a dumbbell in each hand with an underhand and offset grip, so that your thumb is pressed against the outside head of the dumbbell and your palms are facing forward. (Instead of grabbing the dumbbell handle in the middle.) Let the dumbbells hang at arm's length straight down from your shoulders, your palms facing out.

(B) Without moving your upper arms, curl the weights up as high as you can. (Your palms shouldn't turn in during any point in the repetition.)

Pause, then lower the dumbbells back to the starting position.

T-Pushup

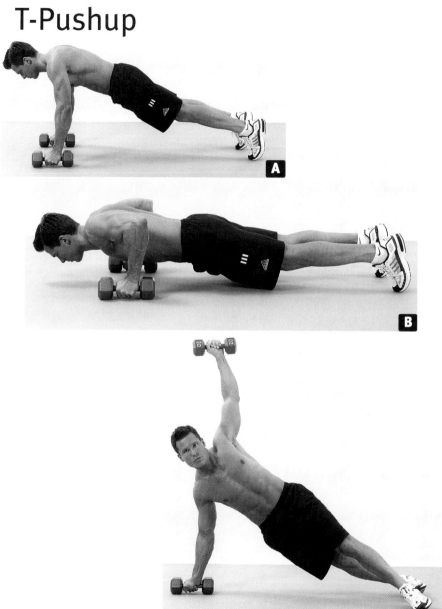

EXERCISE INSTRUCTION

(A) Get into pushup position with your hands on the handles of hexagonal dumb-bells that have been placed shoulder-width apart. Your body should be in a straight line from your shoulders to your ankles.

(B) Lower your chest and then, **(C)** as you come up, rotate your body to raise your right arm and the dumbbell straight up over your shoulder. Your body should form a "T." Lower the dumbbell and your body and repeat with the opposite side.

WORKOUT C

Dynamic Push-up

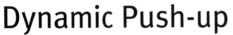

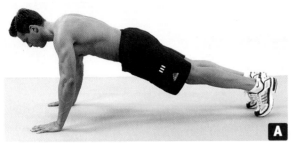

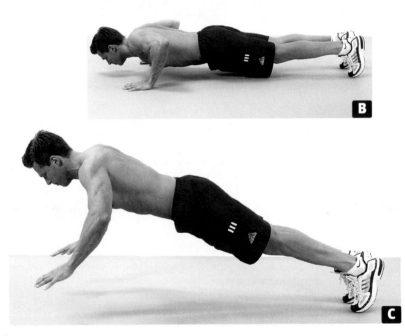

EXERCISE INSTRUCTION

(A) Get into pushup position with your hands slightly wider and in line with your shoulders. Your body should form a straight line from your ankles to your shoulders.

(B) Quickly lower yourself until your upper arms are lower than your elbows,

(C) then forcefully thrust yourself upward until your hands leave the floor. Catch yourself and repeat.

Bench Press

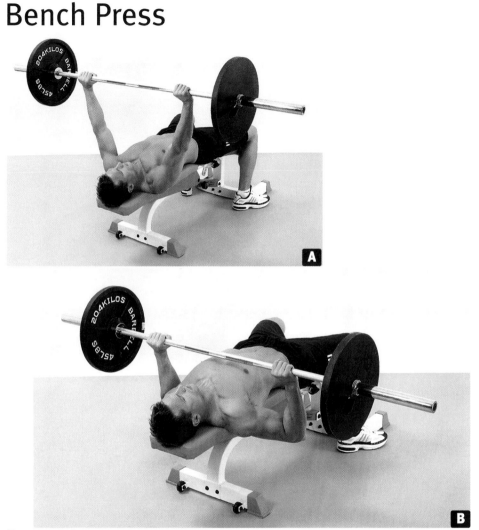

EXERCISE INSTRUCTION

(A) Lie on your back on a flat bench with your feet flat on the floor. Your lower back should be in a naturally arched position; don't flatten it or try to arch it to a greater extent at any time during the lift. Hold a bar with your hands just wider than shoulder-width apart. Lift the bar off the uprights and hold it over your chest at arm's length.

(B) Lower the bar to your chest, keeping your elbows pulled close to your sides (your upper arms will be at about a 45-degree angle to your body in the "down" position). Pause, then push the bar back to the starting position.

WORKOUT C

Chin-up

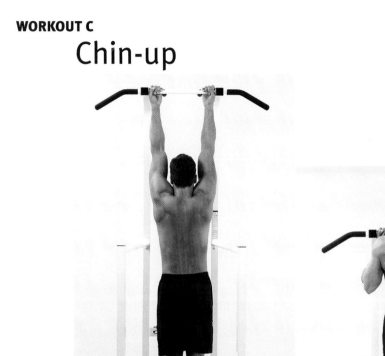

EXERCISE INSTRUCTION

(A) Hang from a chin-up bar with an underhand grip and hands shoulder-width apart. Cross your ankles behind you.

(B) Pull yourself up as high as you can.

Pause and then slowly return to the starting position.

Combo Raise

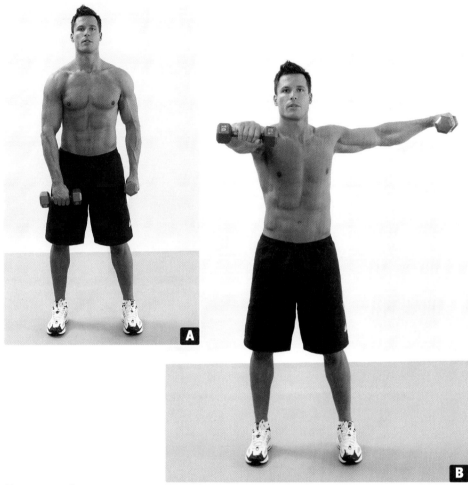

EXERCISE INSTRUCTION

(A) Hold a dumbbell in each hand at arm's length with your elbows slightly bent. Hold the dumbbell in your right hand so that your palm is facing the side of your thigh; hold the dumbbell in your left hand so that your palm is facing the front of your thigh.

(B) Without changing the bend in your elbows, simultaneously raise your right arm out to the side and your left arm out in front of you until they're both parallel to the floor.

Pause, then lower them back to the starting position.

Repeat the movement, but raise your right arm out in front of you and your left arm out to your side. That's one repetition.

Horizontal Lateral Raise

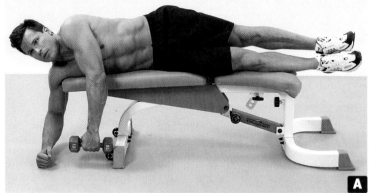

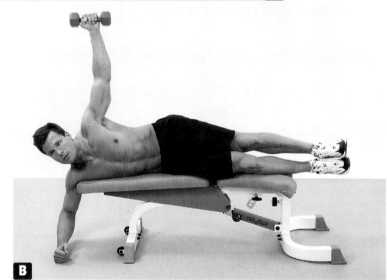

EXERCISE INSTRUCTION

(A) Holding a dumbbell in your right hand, lie on your left side on a flat bench. Let your right arm hang straight down from your body so that it's perpendicular to the floor, your palm turned toward you. Keep your elbow slightly bent.

(B) Without changing the bend in your elbow, raise your arm straight above your shoulder.

Slowly return to the starting position.

Jump Squat

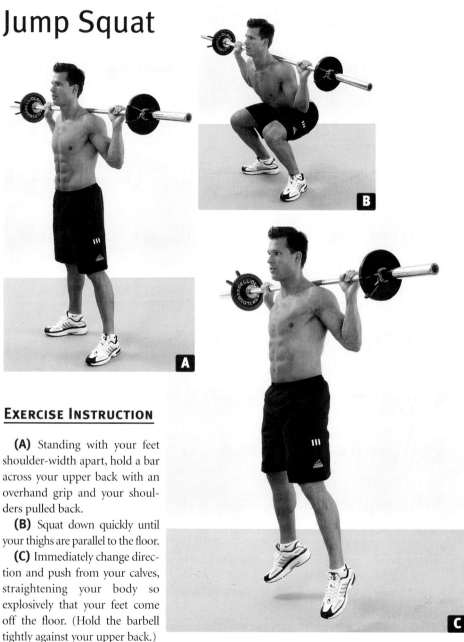

EXERCISE INSTRUCTION

(A) Standing with your feet shoulder-width apart, hold a bar across your upper back with an overhand grip and your shoulders pulled back.

(B) Squat down quickly until your thighs are parallel to the floor.

(C) Immediately change direction and push from your calves, straightening your body so explosively that your feet come off the floor. (Hold the barbell tightly against your upper back.)

Land as softly as possible on your toes, then immediately descend back to the starting position as you shift your weight to your heels and repeat.

Use only the bar in Week 1; add 10 percent of your body weight in Week 2 and another 5 percent (15 percent total) of your body weight in Week 3. So if you weigh 200 pounds, you'll put 20 pounds on the bar in Week 2 and 30 pounds on the bar in Week 3.

WORKOUT D

Bulgarian Split Squat

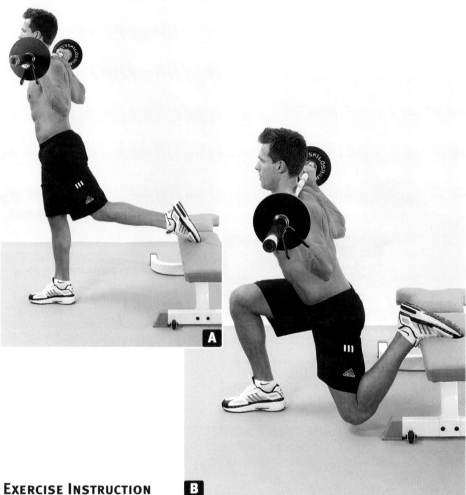

EXERCISE INSTRUCTION

(A) Standing about three feet in front of a bench, hold a barbell with an overhand grip and place it on your upper back (not on your neck). Place your left foot behind you on the bench so that your instep is resting on it.

(B) Lower your body until your front knee is bent 90 degrees and your rear knee nearly touches the floor. Your front lower leg should be perpendicular to the floor and your torso should remain upright.

Push yourself back to the starting position as quickly as you can. Finish all of your repetitions and then repeat the lift, this time with your right foot resting on the bench and your left leg performing the work.

Good Morning

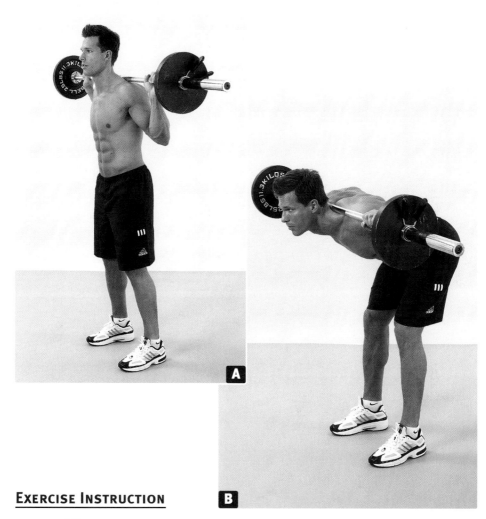

EXERCISE INSTRUCTION

(A) Grab a barbell with an overhand grip and place it so that it rests comfortably across your upper back. Bend your knees slightly.

(B) Slowly bend forward at the hips, maintaining the arch in your lower back as you lower your chest as far as you can or until your upper body is parallel to the floor. Keep your head up and maintain the same angle in your knees throughout the lift.

Pause and then lift your upper body back to the starting position.

WORKOUT D

Lying Dumbbell Triceps Extension

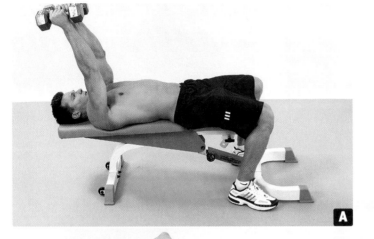

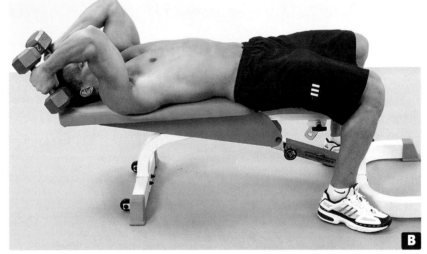

EXERCISE INSTRUCTION

(A) Grab a pair of dumbbells and lie on your back on a flat bench. Hold the dumbbells over your forehead with straight arms, your palms facing each other.

(B) Without moving your upper arms, bend your elbows to lower the dumbbells until your forearms are nearly perpendicular to the floor.

Pause, then lift the weights back to the starting position by straightening your arms.

Barbell Roll-Out

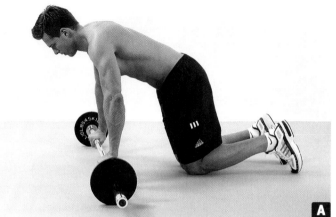

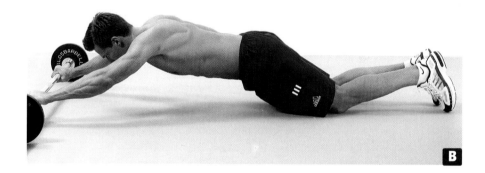

EXERCISE INSTRUCTION

(A) Load a barbell with 10-pound plates on each side and affix collars. Kneel on the floor and grab the bar with an overhand grip, hands shoulder-width apart. In this starting position, your shoulders are over the barbell.

(B) Slowly roll the bar forward, extending your body as far as you can. Use your abdominal muscles to pull the bar back to your knees.

THE WEIGHT WORKOUT
STAGE 2: WEEKS 4 to 6

Warmup: Do two to three circuits of Warmup No. 1 before you do Workout A and Workout C. Do two to three circuits of Warmup No. 2 before you do Workout B and Workout D.

Frequency: Perform each workout once a week, doing Workout A and Workout B on consecutive days, resting a day or two, then completing Workout C and Workout D on consecutive days. So you might do Workout A on Monday, Workout B on Tuesday, Workout C on Thursday and Workout D on Friday.

Exercise Order: Perform each pair of exercises as alternating sets. They're designated as a number and letter pair – for instance, "1A" and "1B," and "2A" and "2B." For each pair, perform one set of the first exercise, rest, then do one set of the second exercise and rest again. Alternate back and forth until you've completed all sets of both exercises.

Rest: Between exercises and sets, rest only as long as it takes for your breathing rate to approach normal. This time period should never exceed two minutes.

REPETITIONS AND WEIGHTS

Workout A: For each exercise, use the repetition and loading scheme below. (It changes each week.) Do as many sets with the prescribed weight as you can. So if you're supposed to do seven repetitions with your seven-repetition maximum (7RM), use the heaviest weight that you can lift seven times without achieving technical failure. That's the weight you'll use for each set. (You'll do fewer sets than you did in Stage 1.) When you achieve technical failure, move on to the next exercise. For each pair of exercises, consider the first, or the "A," exercise your primary exercise (for instance, 1A), and the second, or the "B," exercise your secondary exercise (for instance, 1B). (You'll use a different repetition and loading scheme for each.)

Week 4 Primary Exercise: seven repetitions with your 7RM; **Secondary Exercise:** eight repetitions with your 8RM.

Week 5: Primary Exercise: five repetitions with your 5RM; **Secondary Exercise:** six repetitions with your 6RM.

Week 6: Primary Exercise: three repetitions with your 3RM; **Secondary Exercise:** four repetitions with your 4RM.

FOLLOW THIS RULE OF THUMB ▶
As you lift closer to your one-repetition maximum, you should perform less total volume. That is, the **heavier you lift,** the fewer total sets you do and vice versa

Workout B: For each exercise, use the repetition and loading scheme below. (It changes each week.) Do as many sets with the prescribed weight as you can. So if you're supposed to do 12 repetitions with your 12-repetition maximum (12RM), use the heaviest weight that you can lift 12 times without achieving technical failure. That's the weight you'll use for each set. (You'll do fewer sets than you did in Stage 1.)When you achieve technical failure, move on to the next exercise.

Week 4: 12 repetitions with your 12-repetition maximum.

Week 5: 10 repetitions with your 10-repetition maximum.

Week 6: eight repetitions with your 8-repetition maximum.

Workout C: For each exercise, use the repetition and loading scheme below. (It changes each week.) Do as many sets with the prescribed weight as you can. So if you're supposed to do 12 repetitions with your 12-repetition maximum (12RM), use the heaviest weight that you can lift 12 times without achieving technical failure. That's the weight you'll use for each set. (You'll do fewer sets than you did in Stage 1.)When you achieve technical failure, move on to the next exercise.

Week 4: 12 repetitions with your 12-repetition maximum.

Week 5: 10 repetitions with your 10-repetition maximum.

Week 6: eight repetitions with your 8-repetition maximum.

Workout D: For each exercise, use the repetition and loading scheme below. (It changes each week.) Do as many sets with the prescribed weight as you can. So if you're supposed to do seven repetitions with your seven-repetition maximum (7RM), use the heaviest weight that you can lift seven times without achieving technical failure. That's the weight you'll use for each set. (You'll do fewer sets than you did in Stage 1.)When you achieve technical failure, move on to the next exercise. For each pair of exercises, consider the first, or the "A," exercise your primary exercise (for instance, 1A), and the second, or the "B," exercise your secondary exercise (for instance, 1B). (You'll use a different repetition and loading scheme for each.)

Week 1: Primary Exercise: seven repetitions with your 7RM; **Secondary Exercise:** eight repetitions with your 8RM.

Week 2: Primary Exercise: five repetitions with your 5RM; **Secondary Exercise:** six repetitions with your 6RM.

Week 3: Primary Exercise: three repetitions with your 3RM; **Secondary Exercise:** four repetitions with your 4RM.

ENERGY SYSTEM TRAINING
STAGE 2: WEEKS 4-6
HOW TO DO IT

Do Energy System Training (EST) A on the day following Weight Workout B. Do EST B on the day following Weight Workout D. So you'll perform EST A on Wednesday and EST B on Saturday.

EST A

Week 4: Do eight 15-second sprints at 100 percent of your full effort, resting for 60 seconds between each.

Week 5: Do 10 15-second sprints at 100 percent of your full effort, resting for 60 seconds between each.

Week 6: Do 12 15-second sprints at 100 percent of your full effort, resting for 60 seconds between each.

EST B

Week 4: Do six 30-second sprints at 100 percent of your full effort, resting for 120 seconds between each.

Week 5: Do seven 30-second sprints at 100 percent of your full effort, resting for 120 seconds between each.

Week 6: Do eight 30-second sprints at 100 percent of your full effort, resting for 120 seconds between each.

AT A GLANCE: THE MAXIMUM MUSCLE WORKOUT (STAGE 2)

	Monday	Tuesday	Wednesday	Thursday	Friday	Saturday	Sunday
Week 4	WW A	WW B	EST A	WW C	WW D	EST B	rest
Week 5	WW A	WW B	EST A	WW C	WW D	EST B	rest
Week 6	WW A	WW B	EST A	WW C	WW D	EST B	rest

AT A GLANCE: WORKOUT A (STAGE 2)

EXERCISE	INTENSITY	SETS	REPS
Warmup #1	Bar	2-3	5
1A. Bench Press			
Week 4	7RM	N	7
Week 5	5RM	N	5
Week 6	3RM	N	3
1B. Single-Arm Dumbbell Row			
Week 4	8RM	N	7
Week 5	6RM	N	6
Week 6	4RM	N	4
2A. External Rotation			
Week 4	7RM	N	7
Week 5	5RM	N	5
Week 6	3RM	N	3
2B. Swiss-Ball Crunch			
Week 4	8RM	N	8
Week 5	6RM	N	6
Week 6	4RM	N	4

*N = the number of sets it takes you to reach technical failure

AT A GLANCE: WORKOUT B (STAGE 2)

EXERCISE	INTENSITY	SETS	REPS
Warmup #2	Bar	2-3	5
1A. Elevated-Heels High-Bar Squat			
Week 4	12RM	N	12
Week 5	10RM	N	10
Week 6	8RM	N	8
1B. Weighted Back Extension			
Week 4	12RM	N	12
Week 5	10RM	N	10
Week 6	8RM	N	8
2A. Wide-Grip Barbell Curl			
Week 4	12RM	N	12
Week 5	10RM	N	10
Week 6	8RM	N	8
2B. Incline Dumbbell Triceps Extension			
Week 4	12RM	N	12
Week 5	10RM	N	10
Week 6	8RM	N	8

*N = the number of sets it takes you to reach technical failure

AT A GLANCE: WORKOUT C (STAGE 2)

EXERCISE	INTENSITY	SETS	REPS
Warmup #1	Bar	2-3	5
1A. Neutral-Grip Incline Press			
Week 4	12RM	N	12
Week 5	10RM	N	10
Week 6	8RM	N	8
1B. Chin-up			
Week 4	12RM	N	12
Week 5	10RM	N	10
Week 6	8RM	N	8
2A. Bent-Arm Lateral Raise and Rotation			
Week 4	12RM	N	12
Week 5	10RM	N	10
Week 6	8RM	N	8
2B. Swiss-Ball Side Flexion			
Week 4	12RM	N	12
Week 5	10RM	N	10
Week 6	8RM	N	8

*N = the number of sets it takes you to reach technical failure

AT A GLANCE: WORKOUT D (STAGE 2)

EXERCISE	INTENSITY	SETS	REPS
Warmup #2	Bar	2-3	5
1A. Deadlift			
Week 4	7RM	N	7
Week 5	5RM	N	5
Week 6	3RM	N	3
1B. Single-Leg SBHELC			
Week 4	8RM	N	8
Week 5	6RM	N	6
Week 6	4RM	N	4
2A. Close-Grip Bench Press			
Week 4	7RM	N	7
Week 5	5RM	N	5
Week 6	3RM	N	3
2B. Hammer Curl			
Week 4	8RM	N	8
Week 5	6RM	N	6
Week 6	4RM	N	4

*N = the number of sets it takes you to reach technical failure

Bench Press

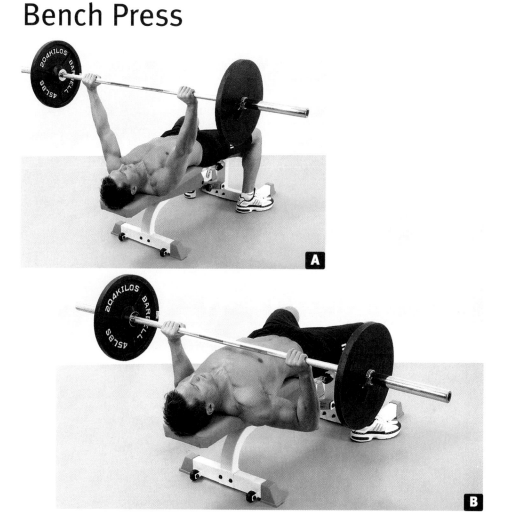

EXERCISE INSTRUCTION

   (A) Lie on your back on a flat bench with your feet flat on the floor. Your lower back should be in a naturally arched position – don't flatten it or try to arch to a greater extent at any time during the lift. Hold the bar with your hands just wider than shoulder-width apart. Lift the bar off the uprights and hold it over your chest at arm's length. **(B)** Lower the bar to your chest, keeping your elbows pulled close to your sides (your upper arms will be at about a 45-degree angle to your body in the "down" position). Pause, then push the bar back to the starting position.

WORKOUT A

Single-Arm Dumbbell Row

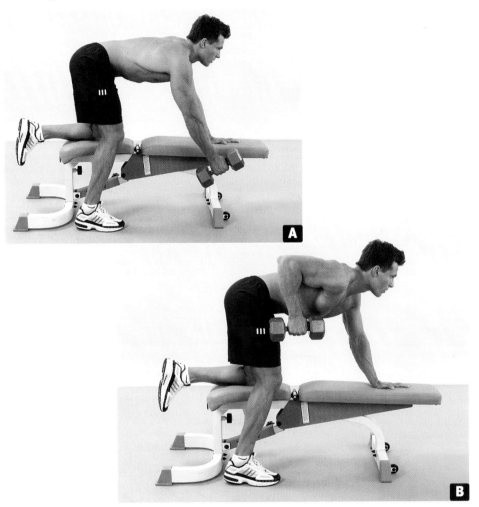

EXERCISE INSTRUCTION

(A) Grab a dumbbell in your right hand and place your left hand and left knee on a flat bench. Keep your back naturally arched and your upper body parallel to the floor. Hold your right arm straight down, but slightly in front of your shoulder. Turn your palm so that it's facing the opposite arm.

(B) Bend your elbow and squeeze your shoulder blade toward the middle of your back, pulling the dumbbell up to the side of your chest and back toward your hip. Keep your elbow close to your body. (Imagine that you're starting a lawn mower.)

Pause and then slowly return to the starting position.

External Rotation

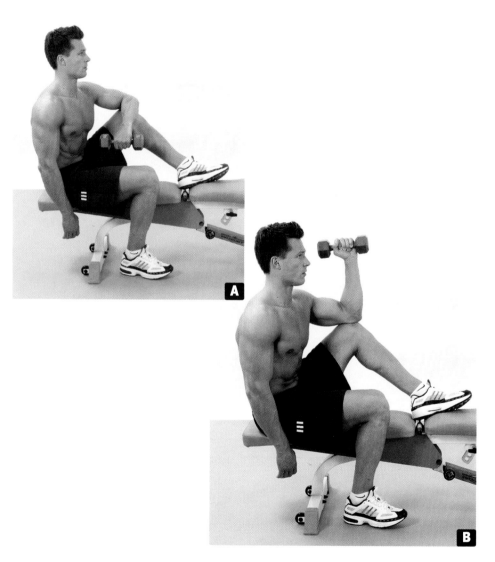

EXERCISE INSTRUCTION

(A) Hold a dumbbell in your left hand and sit on a bench. Place your left foot flat on the bench with your knee bent.

Bend your left elbow 90 degrees and place it on your left knee.

(B) Without changing the bend in your elbow, rotate your upper arm up and back as far as you can. (Your forearm will swing like a gate on hinges.)

Pause, then return to the starting position.

WORKOUT A

Swiss-Ball Crunch

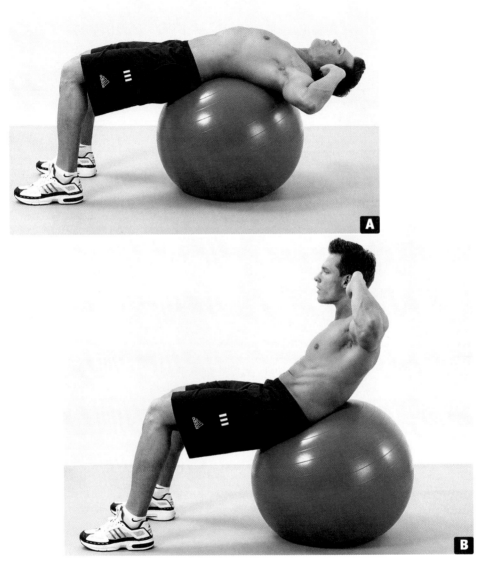

EXERCISE INSTRUCTION

(A) Lie on your back on a Swiss ball, your fingers placed behind your ears. (If that's too easy, hold a weight plate across your chest.)

(B) Raise your head and shoulders and crunch your rib cage toward your pelvis. Pause and slowly return to the starting position.

Elevated Heel High-Bar Squat

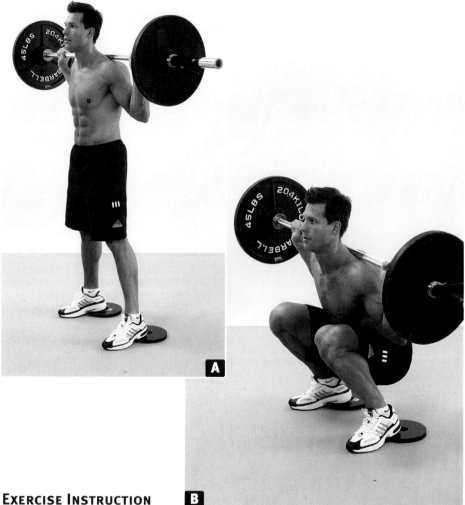

EXERCISE INSTRUCTION

(A) Pull your shoulder blades together and hold a bar with an overhand grip across your upper back. Set your feet set shoulder-width apart and place each heel on a 10-pound weight plate.

(B) Slowly lower your body as far as possible – or until your thighs are at least parallel to the floor – keeping your back naturally arched and your lower legs nearly perpendicular to the floor. Keep your torso as upright as possible.

Pause, then return to the starting position.

WORKOUT B

Weighted Back Extension

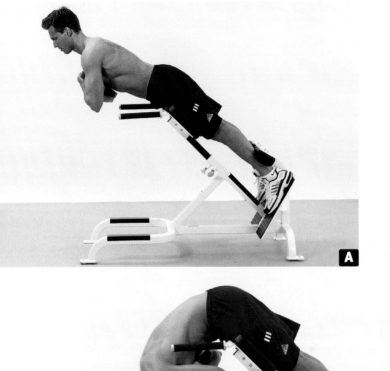

EXERCISE INSTRUCTION

(A) Position yourself in the back-extension station and hook your feet under the leg anchors. Hold a weight across your chest with your arms.

(B) Lower your upper body, allowing your lower back to round until it is just short of being perpendicular to the floor.

Raise your upper body until it is in line with your body and naturally arched.

Wide-Grip Barbell Curl

EXERCISE INSTRUCTION

(A) Grab a barbell with an underhand grip that's slightly wider than shoulder width. Let the bar hang at arm's length in front of your waist, your feet shoulder-width apart.

(B) Curl the bar up as high as you can without moving your upper arms forward.

Pause, then slowly lower the weight to the starting position.

WORKOUT B

Dumbbell Incline Triceps Extension

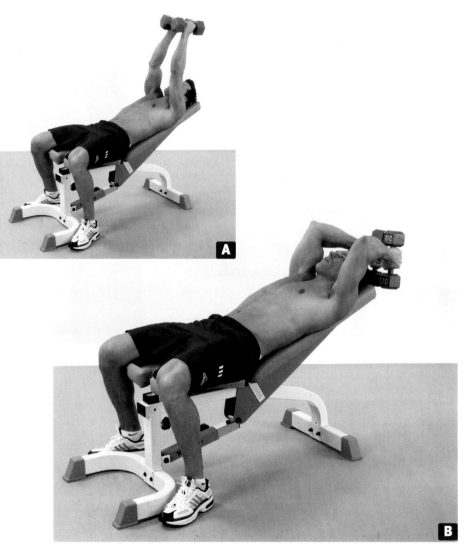

EXERCISE INSTRUCTION

(A) Holding a dumbbell in each hand, lie on your back on an incline bench. Hold the dumbbells over your forehead with straight arms, your palms facing each other.

(B) Without moving your upper arms, bend your elbows to lower the dumbbells until your forearms are nearly perpendicular to the floor.

Pause and then straighten your arms to bring the weights back to the starting position.

Neutral-Grip Incline Press

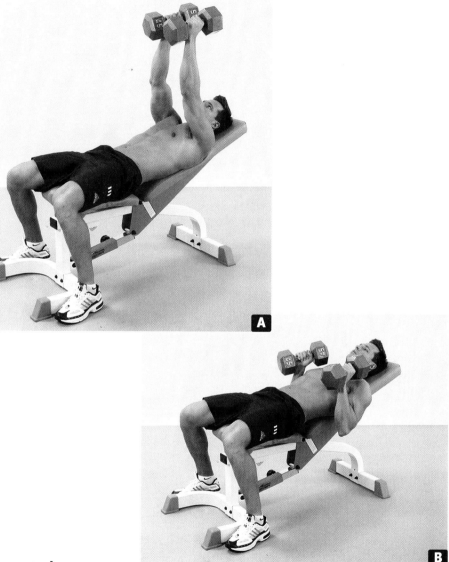

EXERCISE INSTRUCTION

(A) Grab a pair of dumbbells and lie on your back on a bench set to a 15- to 30-degree incline. Lift the dumbbells up at arm's length so they're over your chin and hold them with your palms turned toward each other.

(B) Slowly lower the weights to your upper chest, pause, then push them back up over your chin.

WORKOUT C

Close-Grip Chin-up

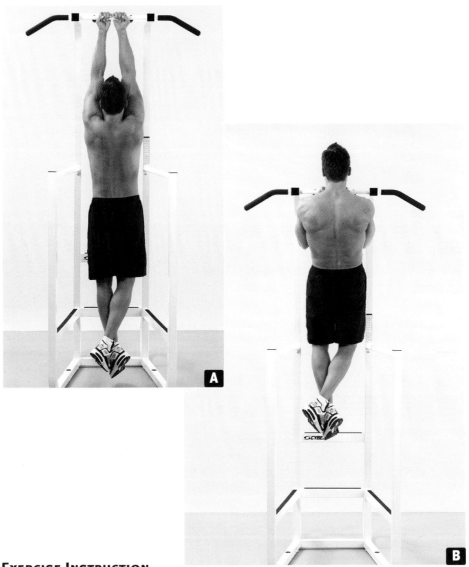

Exercise Instruction

(A) Grab the chin-up-p bar with a shoulder-width, underhand grip. Hang from the bar with your ankles crossed behind you.

(B) Pull yourself up as high as you can.

Pause, then slowly return to the starting position.

Bent-Arm Lateral Raise and Rotation

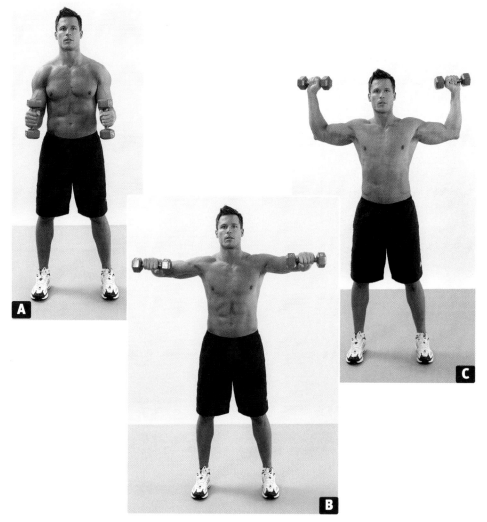

EXERCISE INSTRUCTION

(A) Grab a pair of dumbbells and hold them at arm's length with your palms turned toward each other. Bend your elbows 90 degrees.

(B) Without changing the bend in your elbows, raise your upper arms out to the sides until they're parallel to the floor.

(C) Rotate your upper arm up and back so that your forearm is pointing toward the ceiling.

Pause, then reverse the movement and return to the starting position.

WORKOUT C
Swiss-Ball Side Flexion

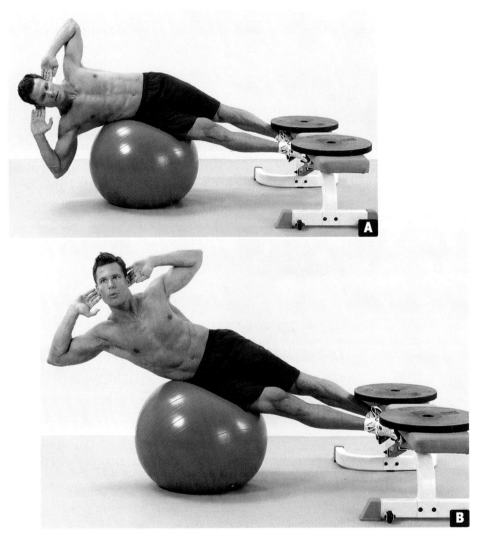

EXERCISE INSTRUCTION

(A) Lie on your side on a Swiss ball and position your feet against a wall or sturdy surface. Place your fingers behind your ears and pull your elbows back as far as you can.

(B) Without moving your hips, raise your upper body as high as you can off the ball.

Pause, then lower yourself back to the starting position.

Deadlift

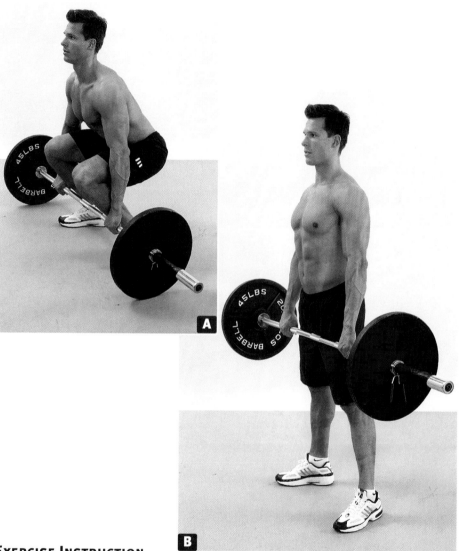

EXERCISE INSTRUCTION

(**A**) Set a barbell on the floor and stand facing it with feet shoulder-width apart. Squat down and grab the barbell with an overhand grip, your hands just outside your legs. Keep your back naturally arched.

(**B**) Without allowing your lower back to round, stand up with the barbell, while pulling your shoulder blades back.

Slowly lower the bar to the starting position.

WORKOUT D

Single-Leg Swiss-Ball Hip Extension and Leg Curl

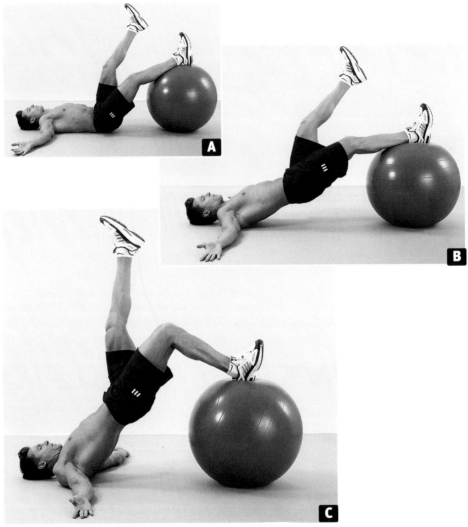

EXERCISE INSTRUCTION

(A) Lie on your back on the floor. Place your left lower leg on a Swiss ball and your right leg in the air, perpendicular to your body. Your hands are facing up, flat on the floor at your sides.

(B) Push your hips up so that your body forms a straight line from your shoulders to your knees.

(C) Without pausing, pull your left heel toward you and roll the ball as close as possible to your butt.

Pause, then reverse the movement and return to the starting position. Finish the repetitions and repeat with your right leg.

Close-Grip Bench Press

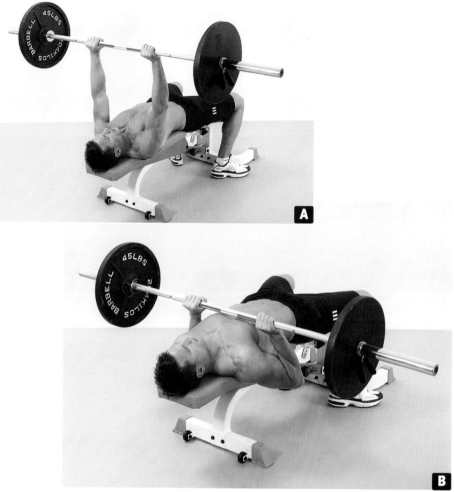

Exercise Instruction

(A) Lie on your back on a flat bench with your feet flat on the floor. Grab the bar with an overhand grip, your hands shoulder-width apart. Hold the bar over your lower chest at arm's length.

(B) Keeping your elbows as close to your torso as possible, slowly lower the bar until it touches your chest.

Pause, then push the bar straight up until your arms are straight and the bar is over your lower chest.

WORKOUT D

Hammer Curl

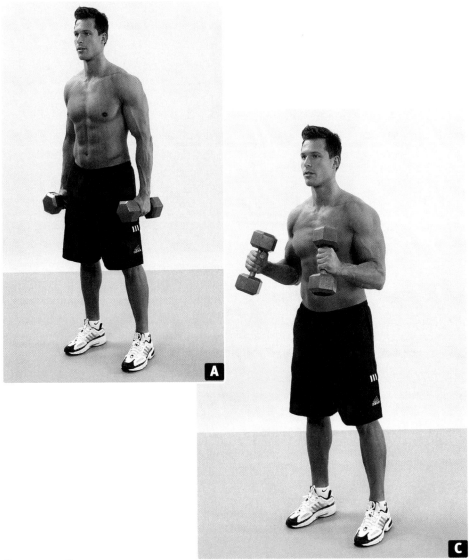

EXERCISE INSTRUCTION

(A) Stand with your feet shoulder-width apart, holding a dumbbell in each hand. Let your arms hang straight down from your shoulders and turn your palms so they're facing each other.

(B) Curl the dumbbells up as high as you can without moving your upper arms forward. Pause, then slowly lower the weights to the starting position.

CHAPTER 5 ▶

Maximum Muscle Diet

HE MAXIMUM MUSCLE DIET IS DESIGNED TO WORK specifically with the Maximum Muscle Workout on page 57. By combining the two plans, you can't fail in your quest to pack on pure muscle – fast.

The diet is simple: You'll eat one gram of protein per pound of body weight and consume 30 percent of your total calories from fat. The remainder of your calories will come from carbohydrates. All of these numbers will vary per person depending on body weight and activity level, which allows you to customize your eating plan. To get started, follow the five-step process described on the next page.

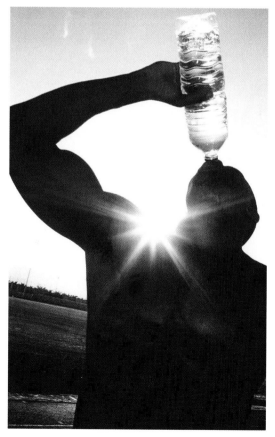

CUSTOMIZE YOUR DIET
Step 1: Calculate Your Total

DAILY CALORIC EXPENDITURE FORMULA		
A. Your weight in pounds		=
B. Multiply A by 11 to get your resting metabolic rate	A x 11	=
C. Multiply B by X* to estimate your caloric expenditure through basic daily activities	B x X	=
D. Strength training: Multiply the number of minutes you lift weight per week by 5:	min. x 5	=
E. Aerobic and sprint training: Multiply the number of minutes per week that you run, cycle or play sports by 8:	min. x 8 =	
F. Add line D and line E, and divide by 7	(D + E)/7 =	
G. Add line C and line F to get your daily caloric needs:	C + F	=
H. Add 500 to line G to get your daily caloric needs to gain one pound per week:	500 + G	= Total

*Determine "X" by choosing your level of daily activity, which is usually dependent on the type of workout do:

Very light (sedentary): X=1.3	Moderate (Some Activity): X=1.7
Light (Office Work): X=1.6	Heavy (Hard labor): X=2.1

Step 2: Calculate Your Protein Amounts

DAILY PROTEIN FORMULA		
I. Your weight in pounds		=
J. Multiply A by 1 to get the total amount of protein in grams that you'll consume daily	A x 1	=
K. Multiply B by 4 to get the total number of calories of protein that you'll consume daily	B x 4	=
L. Divide C by H to get the percentage of your total calories that you'll consume from protein	C / H	= Total

Step 3: Calculate Your Fat Amounts

DAILY FAT FORMULA	
M. Multiply H by 30 percent (.3) to get the total number of calories that you'll consume daily from fat	H x .3 =
N. Divide M by 9 to get the total amount of fat grams that you'll consume daily	M / 9 = Total

Step 4: Calculate Your Carbohydrate Amounts

DAILY CARBOHYDRATE FORMULA	
O. Add K and M	K + M =
P. Subtract O from H to get the total number of calories of carbohydrate that you'll consume daily	H - O =
Q. Divide P by 4 to get the total number of grams of carbohydrate that you'll consume daily	P / 4 =
R. Divide P by H to get the percentage of your total calories that you'll consume from carbohydrates	P / H = Total

Step 5: Gain Muscle

Now that you know how many grams of protein, fat and carbohydrates you need daily, simply design your diet using the guidelines that follow. (For a database of the macronutrient and calorie content of common foods, go to www.fitday.com. You'll find a one-day sample meal plan on the next page.

1. Eat five to six small meals a day. With the exception of your pre- and post-workout nutrition (see No. 4), always eat protein with every meal to keep a steady supply of amino acids available for your body to use for muscle building. Try to divide your calories equally between meals so that you avoid overfueling and increasing your body's propensity to store fat. Shoot for 400 to 700 calories per meal.

2. Avoid "white" foods. You'll still want to become familiar with the glycemic index (see www.glycemicindex.com) and choose the foods that are the lowest. (Technically, low GI foods have a glycemic index of 55 or below.) But we also recommend that you eliminate white bread, white rice, pasta and potatoes, including french fries, potato chips and hash browns. Not all versions of these foods are considered high glycemic, but by following this rule you'll be forced to choose carbohydrates that are higher in fiber and less processed, which will enable you to achieve faster results. (Note: "White" meat is recommended.)

3. Never undereat. If circumstances prevent you from eating "clean," don't skip the meal. For maximizing muscle growth, it's more important to ensure that your body has a surplus of energy than to worry about the kinds of food you are eating. Granted, you want to eat as clean as possible, but if you limit your energy because the right foods aren't available, you'll severely limit your gains. This rule trumps all others when it comes to gaining muscle fast: If worse comes to worst, just eat. And if you're scheduled to eat, but not hungry, eat anyway. Some guys find it tough to consume all of their calories; make sure you do – even if you have to force yourself.

4. Feed your muscles. Your pre- and post-workout nutrition is extremely important. Consider it one of your meals for the day. Here's what to do:

Pre-Workout: Consume 20 grams of protein and 40 grams of carbohydrate immediately before – or immediately before and during – your workout. This will give you ample protein for building muscle, as well as stimulating an increase in insulin to decrease protein breakdown. We recommend that you buy a whey protein supplement for its ease of use and quick digestibility and absorption. (You can eat regular food if that's more convenient: for instance, three ounces of tuna or about five ounces of fat-free turkey.) You need to combine the protein with a high-glycemic carbohydrate (70 and above). Again, you can eat solid food, but we recommend using maltodextrin or dextrose powder. They're complex carbohydrates that quickly raise blood sugar. You can find them at any supplement store and many grocery stores.

Post-Workout: Consume 20 grams of protein and 40 grams of carbohydrates immediately after your workout. Again, regular food is fine, but it's probably not optimal since it's not absorbed into the bloodstream or delivered to the tissues as quickly. For convenience, simply mix together a shake that's 40 grams of protein and 80 grams of carbohydrate. Drink half before your workout and half after your workout. Eat a regular meal or snack within one hour of your workout.

5. Don't worry about gaining fat. Typically, it's probably inevitable to gain some fat as you gain muscle. That's why you'll do the Full-Scale Fat-Loss Phase that follows. So adding some fat is part of the plan, although by eating "clean," you'll minimize the damage, while maximizing your muscle gains.

SAMPLE ONE-DAY MEAL PLAN FOR A 180-POUND GUY

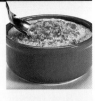

Meal #1
Oatmeal 1 cup (dry)
Raisins 1.5 oz.
Milk (1%) 1 cup
Toasted whole-grain bread, 2 slices / Sugar-free jelly 2 Tbsp.
Carbohydrate 144 grams **Protein** 27 grams **Fat** 10 grams **Calories** 774

Meal #2
Roasted almonds 2 oz.
Plain yogurt 1 cup
Pineapple 1 cup
Carbohydrate 46 grams **Protein** 26 grams **Fat** 36 grams **Calories** 612

Meal #3
Tuna salad 4 oz.
Whole-grain Bread 2 slices
Mayonnaise 1 Tbsp., Relish 1 Tbsp., Tomato 1 slice
Olive oil 1 Tbsp.
Large apple 1 whole
Carbohydrate 88 grams **Protein** 41 grams **Fat** 31 grams **Calories** 795

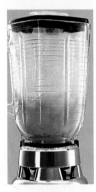

Meal #4
Pre-Workout Shake
Carbohydrate 40 grams **Protein** 20 grams **Fat** 0 grams **Calories** 240

Meal #5
Post-Workout Shake
Carbohydrate 40 grams **Protein** 20 grams **Fat** 0 grams **Calories** 240

Meal #6
Peanut butter 2 Tbsp.
Whole-grain bread, 2 slices
Banana 1/2
Carbohydrate 46 grams **Protein** 14 grams **Fat** 19 grams **Calories** 411

Meal #7
Sirloin 6 oz.
Steamed broccoli 1 cup
Brown rice 1 cup (cooked)
Carbohydrate 49 grams **Protein** 40 grams **Fat** 30 grams **Calories** 626

Daily totals
Calories: 3,698
Carbohydrate: 453 g; 49% of total calories
Protein: 188 g; 20% of total calories
Fat: 126 g; 31% of total calories

CHAPTER 6 ▶

Instant Answers:
Maximum Muscle Phase

THIS SUPPLEMENTAL Q AND A IS DESIGNED to answer common questions about this program, providing more details of how to execute the workouts as well as additional explanation of many of the concepts presented throughout the book.

How do I know if I underestimate my 7- or 12-repetition maximum?

If you use the right method, you shouldn't have to estimate your repetition maximums at all. During each training session of this program you'll use your first "real" set to determine your current repetition maximum. Here's how.

For each exercise, estimate what your repetition maximum will be. (You'll most likely base it on a previous workout or literally make your best guess.) That number won't necessarily be your true 7 or 12RM; you're going to measure it directly. Take the bench press, for example. Let's say in your last bench press workout (before you started the Maximum Muscle Workout) you were able to do 200 pounds for 10 repetitions. So you might estimate your 12RM to be around 190 pounds or so. (There's no need to try to be exact just yet.) Perform your specific warm-up using the ramp-up method (described in Chapter 1) and finish with a weight that approaches 190 pounds. Then start your first "real" set. You'll put 190 pounds on the bar and lift until you achieve technical failure. If you hit technical failure on your 13th repetition, you know that you estimated your 12RM correctly and can start doing sets with the prescribed repetition range (for instance, 10 repetitions in the first week of the Maximum Muscle Workout).

However, suppose you are able to do 14 repetitions before achieving technical failure. That means the weight that you used was too light. Take your rest period, increase the weight slightly and try for your 12 RM again. (The further away you are from you repetition maximum, the more you'll have to increase the weight.) This process should rarely require more than 1 or 2 sets to find your repetition maximum.

You can then continue your training session as prescribed. So if you're doing sets of 10 with your 12RM, you'll then do as many sets as you can without achieving technical failure. Likewise, if you're doing sets of five with your 7RM. As soon as you achieve technical failure, you're done with the exercise.

Testing your repetition maximum each session ensures that you're training at the appropriate intensity each day. The general trend will be a relative increase in weight over the entire training cycle, but don't panic if one day you come into the gym and don't hit at least the same weight as your last training session.

This program adapts to you as an individual. For instance, if you didn't get enough sleep the night before, you just lost your job, your girlfriend left you and your dog died, you may have a little difficulty putting forth your best performance in the gym. That's OK; simply train at the appropriate level for that day.

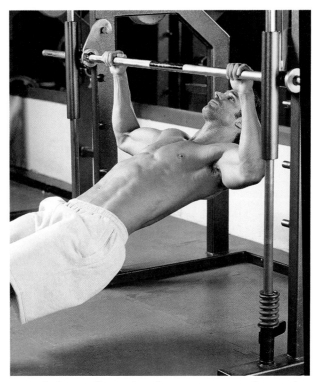

How do I know if I overestimate my 7- or 12-repetition maximum?

Let's use a bench press for example again. Suppose that during your last bench press workout you were able to do 200 pounds for 10 repetitions. So after your warm-up, you start with 190 pounds on the bar and go for 12 repetitions, but hit technical failure on the 11th repetition. That means the weight is too heavy. Take your rest period, reduce the weight slightly and try for your 12RM again. Remember, this process should rarely require more than one or two sets to find your repetition maximum. Otherwise, you're wasting too much energy.

You can then continue your training session as prescribed, completing as many sets with the prescribed number of repetitions as you can and stopping when you achieve technical failure.

How do I know when I should increase the weight?

Weight increases are built right into the training process. By retesting your repetition maximums each training session, your weights will consistently progress upward assuming your nutrition and rest is adequate.

Each time you train, you will perform your first "real" set with your repetition maximum. That maximum is representative of your level of strength and conditioning for that specific day. As you gain strength, your repetition maximums will be higher than the previous training session. This eliminates the guesswork associated with other programs that demand the individual adapt to the program rather than the program adapting to the individual.

Why do we do more reps in the first and third weeks than in the second week?

In the initial week of the Maximum Muscle Workout, the primary goal is to accumulate a volume of work that promotes muscle growth. The second week is a mild intensification week to raise your level of effort as you'll be training a little closer to your true repetition maximum. The higher intensity of effort will promote further "functional" size and strength gains. Although strength will increase, work capacity may decrease due to a reduction in total sets performed. The third week promotes a restoration or even a further increase of work capacity prior to the more intense strength phase that follows in Weeks 4 through 6. You should also notice that your 7RM and the total number of sets you can perform for five repetitions will increase in comparison to the first week.

WHAT DO I DO IF I CAN'T DO THE PRESCRIBED NUMBER OF CHIN-UPS?

GREAT QUESTION. Most programs recommend that you substitute some other form of pulling exercise like a lat pulldown. In our estimation, the lat pulldown is a weak substitute. If you want the V-taper and a muscular back, you've got to do the chin-ups.

That's why we've included a specialized bonus program specifically designed to improve your ability to perform chin-ups. Just substitute the program for your sets of chin-ups in each section of the program. By the time you complete the entire training program, you'll be doing chin-ups with the best of them.

Level 1: You can't do at least one chin-up.

Grab the chin-up bar with a shoulder-width underhand grip and push off a box or bench to help you pull your chin above the bar. Then slowly lower yourself into the hanging position without allowing your movement to accelerate at any point. (You should lower yourself at the same rate from top to bottom.) That's one repetition. Time the duration of your first repetition and record it. Then complete as many repetitions as possible. When your speed of descent accelerates, you're finished with that set. Do two to three sets. (If you're supersetting chin-ups with another exercise, alternate between sets of the two exercises as you normally would. Otherwise, rest for a full two minutes between straight sets.) Each workout, attempt to increase your lowering time up to 30 seconds per repetition. Once you can do one full 30-second repetition, move on to the next level.

Level 2: You can do at least one repetition without significant acceleration (see above) as you lower your body.

Perform one complete repetition without significant acceleration. Rest five to 15 seconds. Perform another repetition. Rest five to 15 seconds. Repeat this process until you can no longer perform a full repetition without increased acceleration of the body. That's one set. Do a total of two sets. (If you're supersetting chin-ups with another exercise, alternate between sets of the two exercises as you normally would. Otherwise, rest for a full two minutes between straight sets.) When you can do four to six repetitions in this manner, move on to the next level.

Level 3: You can perform four to six repetitions without significant acceleration (see above) as you lower your body.

Record the time it takes you to do as many repetitions as possible without significant acceleration as you lower your body. Then rest for that same length of time. Repeat the process until you can no longer complete a full repetition. (You'll do less repetitions and rest for a shorter period each time.) That's one set. Do a total of two sets. (If you're supersetting chin-ups with another exercise, alternate between sets of the two exercises as you normally would, but rest for a full two minutes after the previous exercise. Otherwise, rest for three to five minutes between straight sets.) When you can complete a full set of 12 repetitions without significant acceleration of your lower body, perform the workouts as described.

Why do we do arms on leg day?

Most guys don't understand the best way to train their arms. Typically, they do compound exercises, like presses, rows, dips and chin-ups, and then try to train arms. What happens? You end up having to use "baby weights" to complete your arm workout because your arms are too fatigued from the bigger, heavier, compound exercises.

There's a certain threshold of stimulus from the resistance that is necessary to elicit a gain in strength or size. If you constantly train your arms in a fatigued state, two things will happen: One, you won't gain any size or strength because the weights you're using aren't heavy enough to create sufficient stimulus to do so. Two, you'll expend energy that you could have used for recovery – where the real gains occur – and actually overuse the muscles of your arms, which will eventually make them weaker and smaller.

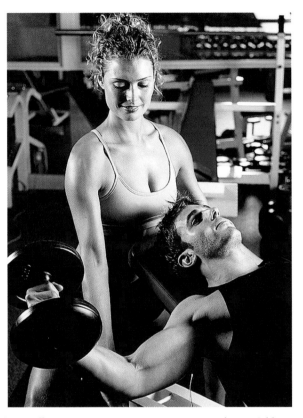

Here's the good part: In general, smaller muscles recover faster than larger ones. By optimizing the volume of training of the larger muscles within this program, we can actually load the arms a little more frequently. We still can't go crazy with too many sets and reps, but with careful application, we can accelerate your gains by performing an arm exercise on the day following the day you perform your heavier pressing and pulling exercises.

Is it OK to take less rest between sets than is recommended?

Only if you're not interested in making any gains in size or strength. Moving too quickly from exercise to exercise prevents sufficient recovery of your nervous system. Truth be told,

your energy systems recover rather quickly – in as little as 30 to 60 seconds. The longer rest periods allow for greater recovery of your nervous system, which keeps the intensity of the exercise high for each subsequent set until you hit the drop off point (technical failure). The more intensity you can maintain during the set, the greater the stimulus for increased size and strength.

Why do we only do four exercises in some workouts? How can that be enough?

Remember this phrase: Do more of less. Most training programs, or the many random "instinctive" programs you see guys performing in the gym, force your body to try to adapt to too many stimuli at once. The body has a limited capacity for what it can adapt to in a specific time period. Every exercise you perform in the gym must be "learned" by the nervous system. As it gets better at performing each exercise, more muscle is recruited and overloaded and therefore strength and size increase.

If you try to perform too many exercises, the nervous system can never learn them effectively enough to increase size and strength. By limiting the number of exercises which the body must adapt to, we maximize the adaptations and accelerate progress.

How come I only do one exercise per muscle group per workout? Don't I need to hit my muscles from different angles?

First, re-read the answer above. Then flip through the rest of the book and you'll see almost 100 different exercises pictured. That's sufficient variation. We've also got variations of loading and exercises throughout the week. Not to be repetitive (OK, maybe a little), but we must limit the number of stimuli to maximize progress.

Why do we do "cardio" if we're trying to gain muscle? Doesn't that burn calories?

It sure does burn calories. So what? You're eating, right? Cardio gets knocked in most size and strength programs, but there's actually a very good reason to do it. Our capacity to recover and tolerate more exercise is based on our overall fitness levels. By avoiding energy system training (aka cardio), as our bodies adapt to the strength training, our overall fitness levels go down. It's simply a function of getting stronger.

Let's make it very simple: The more fit you are, the more stimulus you can tolerate. The more stimulus you can tolerate, the faster and more significant your gains in size and strength.

There's another reason to maintain your energy system training. Keep in mind that this is a complete training program. After a period

of focus on size and strength, we're going to uncover all that new muscle by stripping away the fat. Establishing the foundation of energy system training promotes the formation of

LET'S MAKE IT VERY SIMPLE ►
The more fit you are, the more stimulus you can tolerate. The more stimulus you can tolerate, the faster and more significant your **gains in size** and strength

energy-producing enzymes that you'll use later in the program to eliminate the excess body fat. Avoiding the energy system training during the size and strength phase means that the adaptations later in the program will come slower – or not at all – within the time frame of the program.

If I'm doing supersets and I hit technical failure on one exercise, do I just keep doing the other exercise?

Yes. Each exercise is taken to its individual drop off. If one exercise drops off, the other is continued; you'll just now be doing straight sets for the exercise instead of supersets.

How do I know if I'm eating enough calories?

You should be gaining a pound a week. The day you start the plan, weigh yourself in the morning, after you've gone to the restroom, but before you eat breakfast. The following week, weigh yourself again, following the same procedure. If you haven't gained one pound, increase your calorie intake by 250 calories a day. Continue this process each week until you're gaining at least a pound a week. In this case, it's better to err on the side of gaining more than less. You'll take any extra fat off during the Full-Scale Fat-Loss phase.

PART III

FULL-SCALE FAT-LOSS PHASE

CHAPTER 7 ▶

Full-Scale Fat-Loss Workout

THIS SIX-WEEK CYCLE INCLUDES TWO PARTS: weight training and energy system training. Follow the directions for each. Combine this workout plan with the Full-Scale Fat-Loss Diet on page 139.

THE WEIGHT WORKOUT
STAGE 1: WEEKS 1 to 3

Warm-up: Before each workout, do two to three circuits of either Warmup No. 1 or Warmup No. 2 (your choice). Perform your ramp-up warm-up as described in Chapter 1 prior to the appropriate exercises.

Frequency: Perform each workout once a week, resting at least a day between each. So you might do Workout A on Monday, Workout B on Wednesday and Workout C on Friday.

Exercise Order: Perform the exercises using one of two techniques: straight sets or supersets. Straight sets are designated simply as a number – for instance, "2" or "5." Supersets are designated as a number and letter pair – for instance, "1A" and "1B." For straight sets, complete all sets of that exercise – resting between each set – before moving on to the next. For supersets, perform one set of the first exercise, then immediately do one set of the second exercise before resting for the prescribed amount of time. Repeat until you've completed all sets of both exercises, then move on to the next pair of exercises.

Rest: Between sets and exercises, rest only as long as it takes for your breathing rate to approach normal. This time period should never exceed two minutes.

Repetitions and Weights

Workout A: Perform this workout as supersets. For each exercise, use a weight that's equal to your six-repetition maximum. (The heaviest weight you can lift six times without achieving technical failure.) Do three sets of each exercise, resting only as long it takes for your breathing to return to normal between supersets. Never rest for more than two minutes.

Workout B: Perform this workout as supersets. For each exercise, use a weight that's equal to your 20-repetition maximum. (The heaviest weight you can lift 20 times without achieving technical failure.) Do two sets of each exercise, resting only as long as it takes for your breathing to return to normal between supersets. (Limit this time period to two minutes, regardless.)

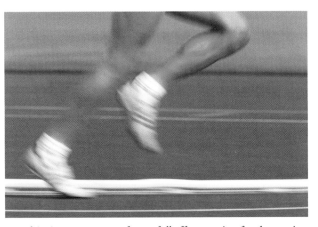

Workout C: Perform this workout as a circuit. For each exercise, use a weight that's equal to your 12-repetition maximum. (The heaviest weight you can lift 12 times without achieving technical failure.) Do a total of four circuits, resting only as long it takes for your breathing to return to normal between circuits. (Limit this time period to two minutes, regardless.)

ENERGY SYSTEM TRAINING
STAGE 1: WEEKS 1 to 3
HOW TO DO IT

Do Energy System Training (EST) A on the day following Weight Workout A, EST B on the day following Weight Workout B and EST C on the day following Weight Workout C. So you might perform EST A on Tuesday, EST B on Thursday and EST C on Saturday.

EST A

Week 1: Do five 60-second sprints at 100 percent of your full effort, resting for three minutes between each.

Week 2: Do six 60-second sprints at 100 percent of your full effort, resting for three minutes between each.

Week 3: Do seven 60-second sprints at 100 percent of your full effort, resting for three minutes between each.

EST B

Week 1: Do 10 30-second sprints at 100 percent of your full effort, resting for 90 seconds between each.

Week 2: Do 11 30-second sprints at 100 percent of your full effort, resting for 90 seconds between each.

Week 3: Do 12 30-second sprints at 100 percent of your full effort, resting for 90 seconds between each.

EST C

Week 1: Do five 60-second sprints at 100 percent of your full effort, resting for three minutes between each.

Week 2: Do six 60-second sprints at 100 percent of your full effort, resting for three minutes between each.

Week 3: Do seven 60-second sprints at 100 percent of your full effort, resting for three minutes between each.

AT A GLANCE: THE FULL-SCALE FAT LOSS WORKOUT (STAGE 1)

	Monday	Tuesday	Wednesday	Thursday	Friday	Saturday	Sunday
Week 1	WW A	EST A	WW B	EST B	WW C	EST C	rest
Week 2	WW A	EST A	WW B	EST B	WW C	EST C	rest
Week 3	WW A	EST A	WW B	EST B	WW C	EST C	rest

AT A GLANCE: WORKOUT A (STAGE 1)

EXERCISE	INTENSITY	SETS	REPS
Warmup #1	Bar	2-3	5
1A. Dumbbell Alternating Lunge			
Week 1	6RM	3	6
Week 2	6RM	3	6
Week 3	6RM	3	6
1B. Squat			
Week 1	6RM	3	6
Week 2	6RM	3	6
Week 3	6RM	3	6
2A. Incline Dumbbell Fly			
Week 1	6RM	3	6
Week 2	6RM	3	6
Week 3	6RM	3	6
2B. Incline Dumbbell Press			
Week 1	6RM	3	6
Week 2	6RM	3	6
Week 3	6RM	3	6
3A. Rear Lateral Raise			
Week 1	6RM	3	6
Week 2	6RM	3	6
Week 3	6RM	3	6
3B. Bent-over Row			
Week 1	6RM	3	6
Week 2	6RM	3	6
Week 3	6RM	3	6

*N = the number of sets it takes you to reach technical failure

AT A GLANCE: WORKOUT C (STAGE 1)

EXERCISE	INTENSITY	SETS	REPS
Warmup #1	Bar	2-3	5
1A. Wide-stance Squat			
Week 1	12RM	4	12
Week 2	12RM	4	12
Week 3	12RM	4	12
1B. Dumbbell Bench Press			
Week 1	12RM	4	12
Week 2	12RM	4	12
Week 3	12RM	4	12
1C. Wide-grip Chin-up			
Week 1	12RM	4	12
Week 2	12RM	4	12
Week 3	12RM	4	12
1D. Push Press			
Week 1	12RM	4	12
Week 2	12RM	4	12
Week 3	12RM	4	12

*N = the number of sets it takes you to reach technical failure

AT A GLANCE: WORKOUT B (STAGE 1)

EXERCISE	INTENSITY	SETS	REPS
Warmup #2	Bar	2-3	5
1A. Dumbbell Squat			
Week 1	20RM	2	20
Week 2	20RM	2	20
Week 3	20RM	2	20
1B. Swiss-ball Reverse Hyperextension			
Week 1	20RM	2	20
Week 2	20RM	2	20
Week 3	20RM	2	20
2A. Pushup			
Week 1	20RM	2	20
Week 2	20RM	2	20
Week 3	20RM	2	20
2B. Underhand-grip Inverted Row			
Week 1	20RM	2	20
Week 2	20RM	2	20
Week 3	20RM	2	20
3A. Neutral-grip Shoulder Press			
Week 1	20RM	2	20
Week 2	20RM	2	20
Week 3	20RM	2	20
3B. Incline Reverse Crunch			
Week 1	20RM	2	20
Week 2	20RM	2	20
Week 3	20RM	2	20
4A. Dumbbell Curl			
Week 1	20RM	2	20
Week 2	20RM	2	20
Week 3	20RM	2	20
4B. Triceps Kickback			
Week 1	20RM	2	20
Week 2	20RM	2	20
Week 3	20RM	2	20

*N = the number of sets it takes you to reach technical failure

WORKOUT A

Dumbbell Alternating Lunge

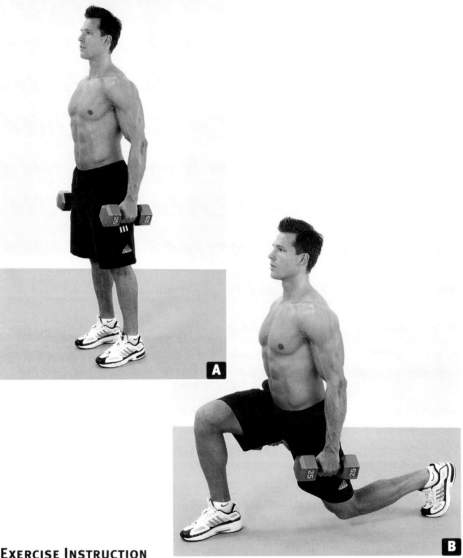

EXERCISE INSTRUCTION

(A) Grab a pair of dumbbells and hold them at your sides. Stand with your feet hip-width apart.

(B) Step forward with your left leg and lower your body until your front knee is bent 90 degrees and your rear knee nearly touches the floor. Your front lower leg should be perpendicular to the floor and your torso should remain upright.

Push yourself back up to the starting position as quickly as you can and repeat with your right leg. That's one repetition.

Squat

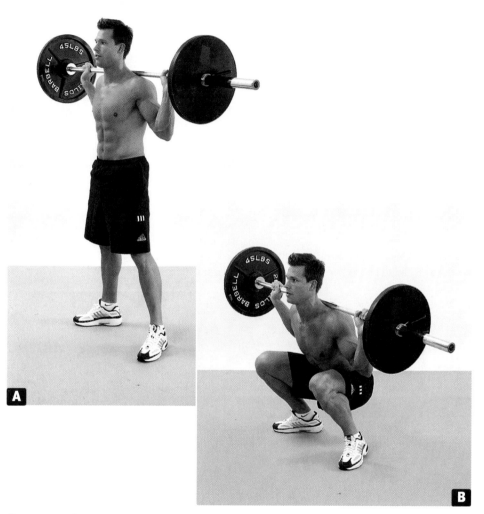

EXERCISE INSTRUCTION

(A) Hold a bar across your upper back with an overhand grip, your feet are shoulder-width apart and your shoulders are pulled back.

(B) Slowly lower your body as far as possible – or until your thighs are at least parallel to the floor – keeping your back naturally arched and your lower legs nearly perpendicular to the floor.

Pause, then return to the starting position.

WORKOUT A

Incline Dumbbell Fly

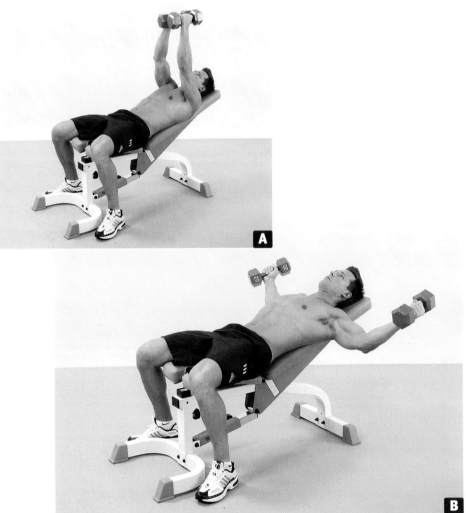

EXERCISE INSTRUCTION

(A) Holding a dumbbell in each hand, lie on your back on a bench set to a 15- to 30-degree incline. Lift the dumbbells and hold them over your chest with your elbows slightly bent and your palms facing each other.

(B) Slowly lower the dumbbells down and slightly back until your upper arms are parallel to the floor and in line with your ears.

Pause, then lift the dumbbells back to the starting position.

Incline Dumbbell Press

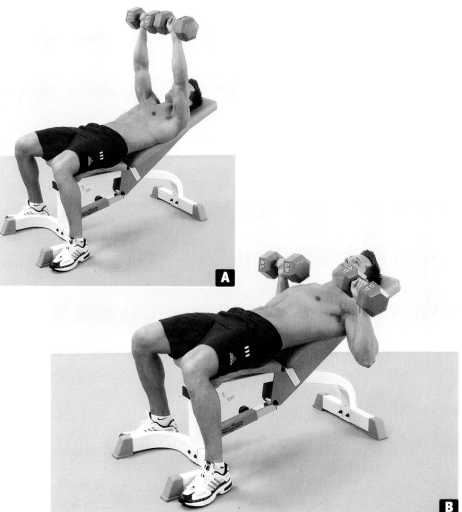

EXERCISE INSTRUCTION

(**A**) Holding a dumbbell in each hand, lie on your back on a bench set to a 15- to 30-degree incline. Lift the dumbbells up at arm's length so they're over your chin and hold them with your palms turned toward your feet so that your thumbs are facing each other.

(**B**) Slowly lower the weights to your upper chest, pause, then push them back up.

WORKOUT A
Rear Lateral Raise

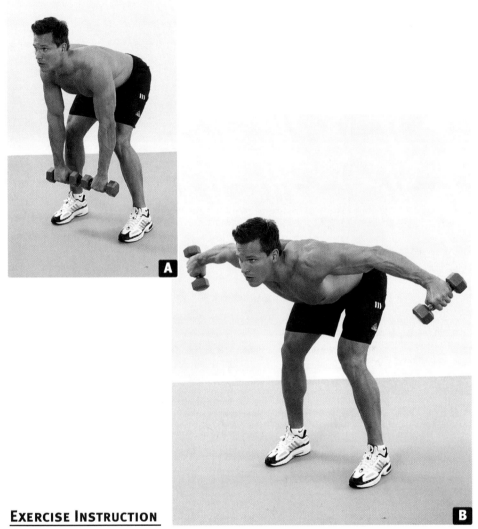

EXERCISE INSTRUCTION

(A) Grab a pair of dumbbells with an overhand grip and hold them at your side, your elbows slightly bent. Stand with your feet shoulder-width apart and knees slightly bent. Bend at the hips, keeping your back naturally arched, and lower your torso until it's almost parallel to the floor. Let the dumbbells hang straight down from your shoulders.

(B) Raise the dumbbells as high as you can without changing the bend in your elbows.

Pause, then lower the dumbbells to the starting position.

Bent-over Row

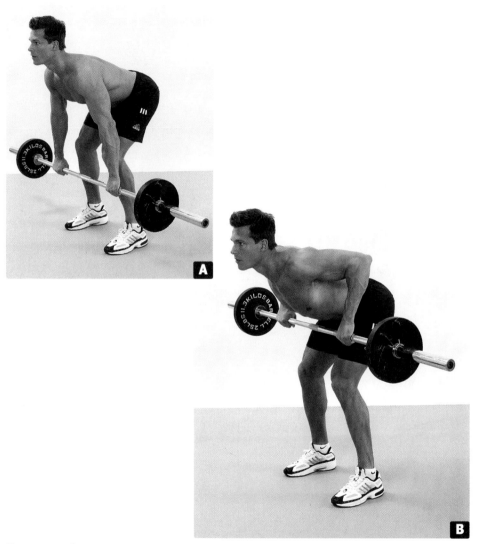

EXERCISE INSTRUCTION

(A) Grab a barbell with an overhand grip that's just beyond shoulder-width and hold it at arm's length. Stand with your feet shoulder-width apart and knees slightly bent. Bend at the hips, keeping your lower back naturally arched, and lower your torso until it's almost parallel to the floor. Let the bar hang straight down from your shoulders.

(B) Pull the bar up to your torso, pause, then slowly lower it.

WORKOUT B

Dumbbell Squat

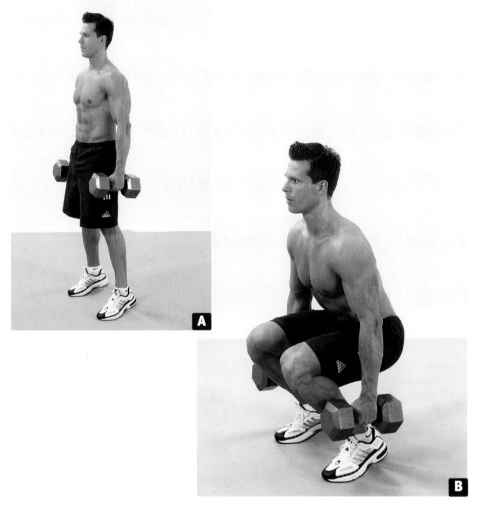

EXERCISE INSTRUCTION

(A) Hold a dumbbell in each hand at arm's length at your sides. Set your feet shoulder-width apart.

(B) Slowly lower your body as far as possible – or until your thighs are at least parallel to the floor – keeping your back naturally arched and your lower legs nearly perpendicular to the floor.

When your upper thighs are parallel to the floor, pause and then return to the starting position.

Swiss-Ball Reverse Hyperextension

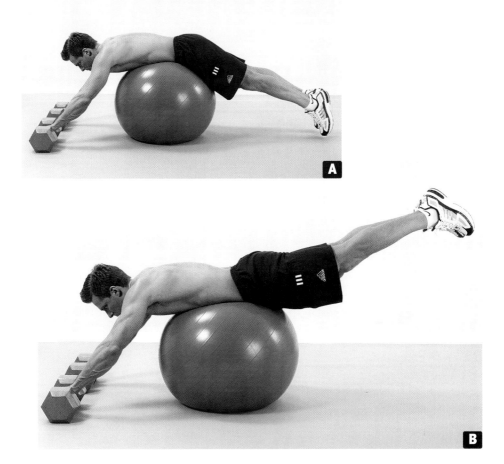

EXERCISE INSTRUCTION

(A) Place a pair of heavy dumbbells in front of a Swiss ball. Lie chest down on the ball and hold the dumbbells for stability. Position your body so that your abdomen is resting on top of the ball . Keep your legs together and nearly straight.

(B) Without changing the bend in your knees, lift your hips and thighs until they're in line with your torso.

Pause, then lower your legs until your feet nearly touch the floor. That's one repetition.

WORKOUT C

Push-up

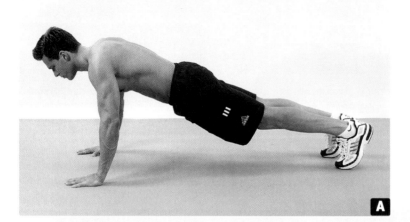

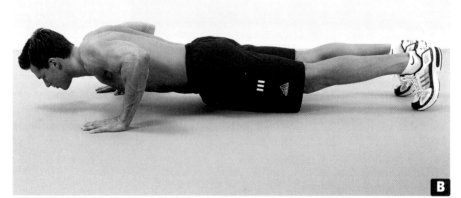

EXERCISE INSTRUCTION

    (A) Get into push-up position – your hands set slightly wider than and in line with your shoulders – with your arms straight.

    (B) Without allowing your hips to sag, lower your body until your chest nearly touches the floor.

    Pause, then push yourself back up to the starting position.

Underhand-Grip Inverted Row

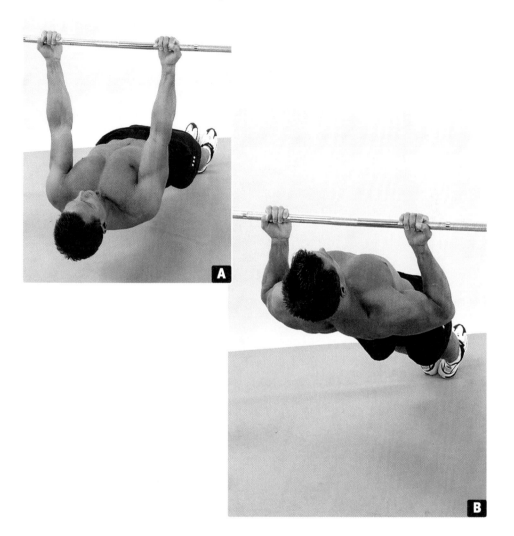

EXERCISE INSTRUCTION

(A) Secure a bar 3 to 4 feet above the floor (a Smith machine works well). Position yourself under the bar and grab it with a shoulder-width, underhand grip. Hang at arm's length from the bar with your body straight in a straight line from your ankles to your shoulders.

(B) Keeping your body rigid, pull your chest to the bar.

Pause, then lower yourself back to the starting position.

WORKOUT B

Neutral-Grip Shoulder Press

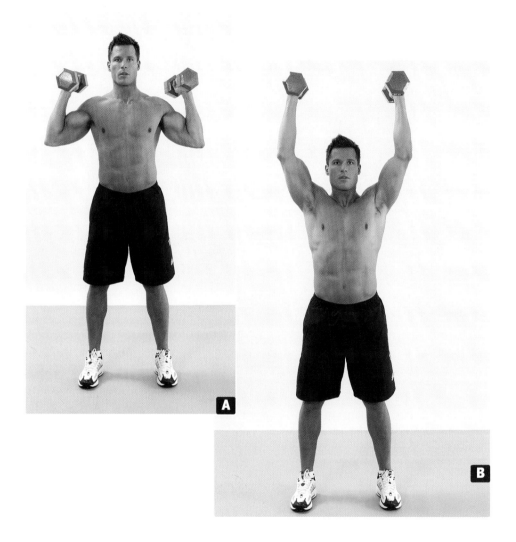

EXERCISE INSTRUCTION

(A) Standing with your feet shoulder-width apart, hold a dumbbell in each hand. Bend your arms so that the dumbbells are just outside of your shoulders and your palms are facing each other.

(B) Push the weights directly above your shoulders until your arms are straight, then slowly lower them.

Incline Reverse Crunch

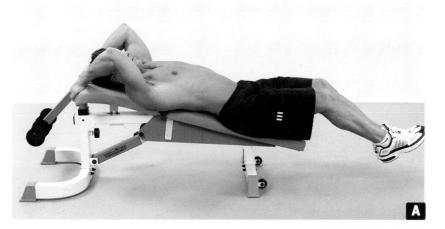

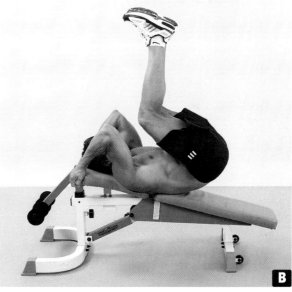

EXERCISE INSTRUCTION

(A) Lie on a slant board with your hips lower than your head and your knees slightly bent.

(B) Pull your hips upward and inward, as if you were emptying a bucket of water that's resting on your pelvis. Keep your knees at the same angle throughout the movement.

Pause, then slowly lower your hips to the starting position.

Note: If this exercise is too challenging, simply perform it on the floor.

WORKOUT B

Dumbbell Curl

A

B

EXERCISE INSTRUCTION

(A) Grab a pair of dumbbells with an underhand grip and hold them at arm's length beside your thighs. Stand straight with your upper arms tucked against your sides. Your feet should be shoulder-width apart, knees slightly bent.

(B) Curl the dumbbells toward your chest as far as you can while keeping your upper arms still.

Pause, then slowly return to the starting position.

Triceps Kickback

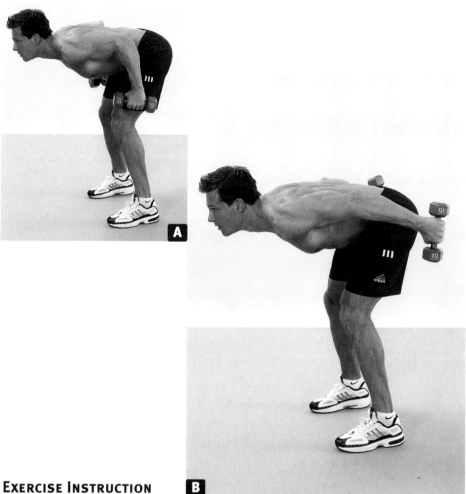

EXERCISE INSTRUCTION

(A) Grab a pair of dumbbells and stand with your feet shoulder-width apart and your knees slightly bent. Maintaining the natural arch in your back, bend at the hips and lower your torso until it's almost parallel to the floor. Bend your elbows 90 degrees and raise your upper arms so that they're parallel to the floor and as close to your torso as possible, your palms facing each other.

(B) Without moving your upper arms, lift your lower arms until your elbows lock.

Pause, then lower the dumbbells to the starting position.

WORKOUT C

Wide-Stance Squat

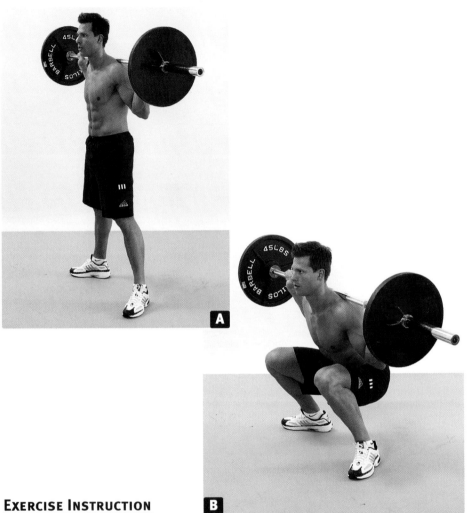

EXERCISE INSTRUCTION

(A) Hold a bar across your upper back with an overhand grip. Set your feet about twice shoulder-width apart, your toes pointing slightly out.

(B) Slowly lower your body as far as possible – or until your thighs are at least parallel to the floor – keeping your back naturally arched and your lower legs nearly perpendicular to the floor.

Pause and then return to the starting position.

Dumbbell Bench Press

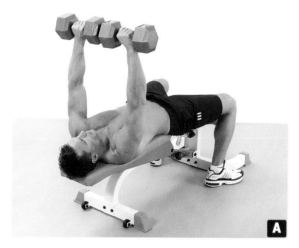

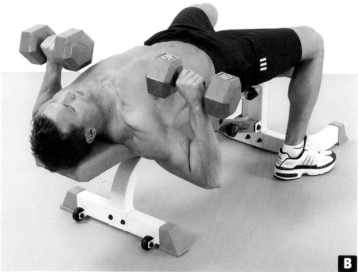

EXERCISE INSTRUCTION

(A) Grab a pair of dumbbells and lie on your back on a flat bench, holding the dumbbells over your chest.

(B) Lower the dumbbells to the sides of your chest, pause, then push them back up the starting position.

WORKOUT C

Wide-Grip Chin-Up

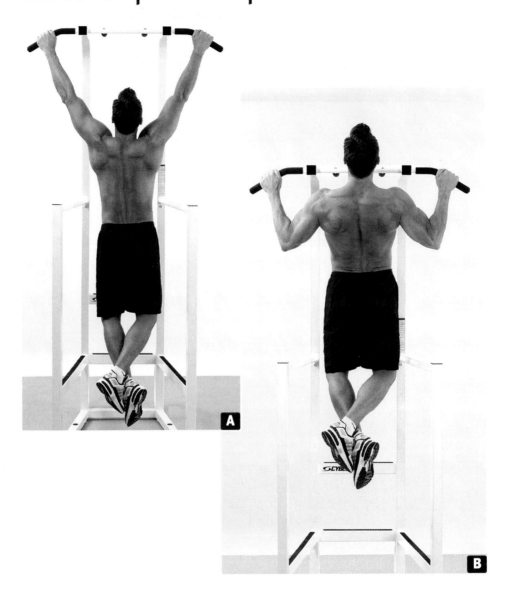

EXERCISE INSTRUCTION

(A) Grab the chin-up bar with an overhand grip that's twice your shoulder width; cross your ankles behind you and hang.

(B) Pull yourself up as high as you can.

Pause, then slowly return to the starting position.

Push Press

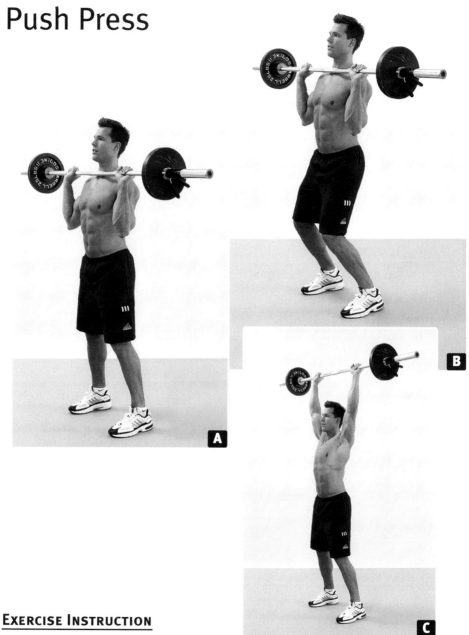

EXERCISE INSTRUCTION

    (A) Standing with your feet shoulder-width apart and knees slightly bent, hold a barbell with a shoulder-width, overhand grip

    (B) Dip your knees slightly and push up with your legs as you press the barbell over your head.

    (C) Keeping your torso upright, lean your head back slightly as you push the barbell above you. Lower the barbell to the starting position.

THE WEIGHT WORKOUT
STAGE 2: WEEKS 4 to 6

Warm-up: Before each workout, do two to three circuits of either Warm-up No. 1 or Warm-up No. 2 (your choice). (Perform your ramp-up warm-up as described in Chapter 1 prior to the appropriate exercises.)

Frequency: Perform each workout once a week, resting at least a day between each. So you might do Workout A on Monday, Workout B on Wednesday and Workout C on Friday.

Exercise Order: Perform all of the exercises in each workout as straight sets. So you'll complete all sets of the first exercise – resting between each set – before moving on to the second.

Rest: Between sets and exercises, rest until you feel completely recovered. As a general guide, it will be about three to five minutes.

REPETITIONS AND WEIGHTS

Perform all of the exercises in each workout as straight sets. For each exercise, use the heaviest weight that allows you to perform at least four but no more than six repetitions before achieving technical failure. So you'll be using your four- to six-repetition maximum. Then do as many sets with that weight as you can. When you achieve technical failure on your fourth or earlier repetition, move on to the next exercise.

ENERGY SYSTEM TRAINING
STAGE 2: WEEKS 4 to 6

Do Energy System Training (EST) A on the day following Weight Workout A, EST B on the day following Weight Workout B and EST C on the day following Weight Workout C. So you might perform EST A on Tuesday, EST B on Thursday, and EST C on Saturday.

EST A

Week 4: Do eight 60-second sprints at 100 percent of your full effort, resting for two minutes between each.

Week 5: Do nine 60-second sprints at 100 percent of your full effort, resting for two minutes between each.

Week 6: Do 10 60-second sprints at 100 percent of your full effort, resting for two minutes between each.

EST B

Week 4: Do 13 30-second sprints at 100 percent of your full effort, resting for 60 seconds between each.

Week 5: Do 14 30-second sprints at 100 percent of your full effort, resting for 60 seconds between each.

Week 6: Do 15 30-second sprints at 100 percent of your full effort, resting for 60 seconds between each.

EST C

Week 4: Do eight 60-second sprints at 100 percent of your full effort, resting for two minutes between each.

Week 5: Do nine 60-second sprints at 100 percent of your full effort, resting for two minutes between each.

Week 6: Do 10 60-second sprints at 100 percent of your full effort, resting for two minutes between each.

AT A GLANCE: THE FULL-SCALE FAT-LOSS WORKOUT (STAGE 2)

	Monday	Tuesday	Wednesday	Thursday	Friday	Saturday	Sunday
Week 4	WW A	EST A	WW B	EST B	WW C	EST C	rest
Week 5	WW A	EST A	WW B	EST B	WW C	EST C	rest
Week 6	WW A	EST A	WW B	EST B	WW C	EST C	rest

AT A GLANCE: WORKOUT A (STAGE 2)

EXERCISE	INTENSITY	SETS	REPS
Warmup #1	Bar	2-3	5
1A. Snatch-Grip Deadlift			
Week 4	4-6RM	N	4-6
Week 5	4-6RM	N	4-6
Week 6	4-6RM	N	4-6
1B. Push Press			
Week 4	4-6RM	N	4-6
Week 5	4-6RM	N	4-6
Week 6	4-6RM	N	4-6

*N = the number of sets it takes you to reach technical failure

AT A GLANCE: WORKOUT B (STAGE 2)

EXERCISE	INTENSITY	SETS	REPS
Warmup #1	Bar	2-3	5
1. Bench Press			
Week 4	4-6RM	N	4-6
Week 5	4-6RM	N	4-6
Week 6	4-6RM	N	4-6
2. Barbell Curl			
Week 4	4-6RM	N	4-6
Week 5	4-6RM	N	4-6
Week 6	4-6RM	N	4-6

*N = the number of sets it takes you to reach technical failure

AT A GLANCE: WORKOUT C (STAGE 2)

EXERCISE	INTENSITY	SETS	REPS
Warmup #1	Bar	2-3	5
1. Chin-up			
Week 4	4-6RM	N	4-6
Week 5	4-6RM	N	4-6
Week 6	4-6RM	N	4-6
2. Dip			
Week 4	4-6RM	N	4-6
Week 5	4-6RM	N	4-6
Week 6	4-6RM	N	4-6

*N = the number of sets it takes you to reach technical failure

WORKOUT A

Snatch-Grip Deadlift

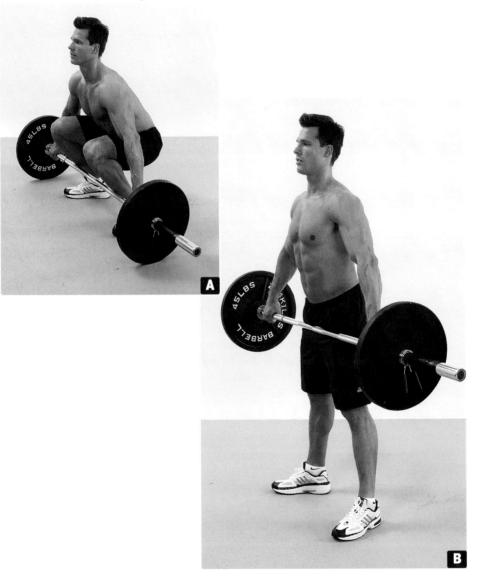

EXERCISE INSTRUCTION

(A) Set a barbell on the floor and stand facing it. Squat down and grab it with an overhand grip, your hands spaced about twice shoulder-width apart. Keep your back naturally arched.

(B) Without allowing your lower back to round, stand up with the barbell, pulling your shoulder blades back.

Slowly lower the bar to the starting position.

Push Press

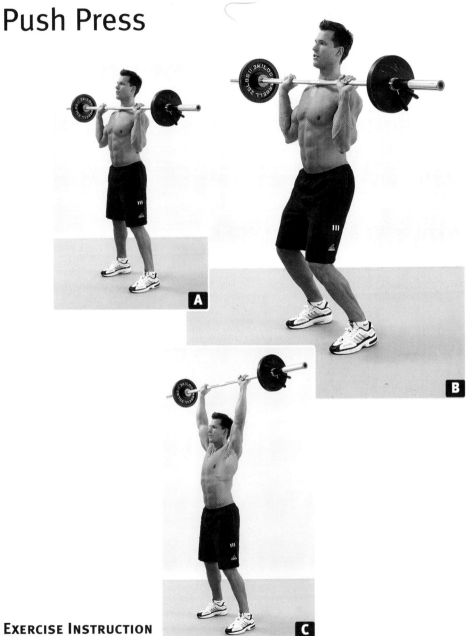

EXERCISE INSTRUCTION

(A) Grab a barbell with a shoulder-width, overhand grip. Stand holding the barbell at shoulder level, your feet shoulder-width apart and knees slightly bent.

(B) Dip your knees slightly and push up with your legs as you press the barbell over your head. Lean your head back slightly as you push the barbell above you, but keep your torso upright.

Lower the bar to the starting position.

WORKOUT B

Bench Press

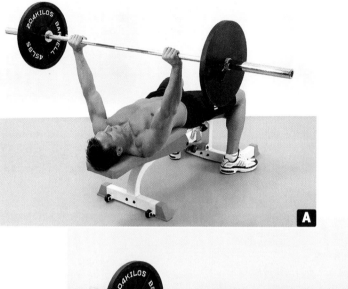

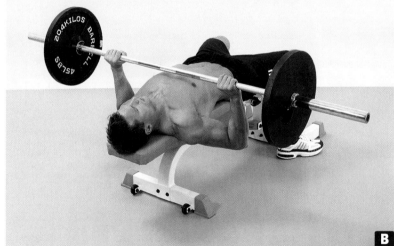

EXERCISE INSTRUCTION

(A) Lie on your back on a flat bench with your feet flat on the floor. Your lower back should be in a naturally arched position – don't flatten it or try to arch to a greater extent at any time during the lift. Hold the bar with your hands just wider than shoulder-width apart. Lift the bar off the uprights and hold it over your chest.

(B) Lower the bar to your chest, keeping your elbows pulled close to your sides (your upper arms will be at about a 45-degree angle to your body in the "down" position).

Pause, then push the bar back to the starting position.

Barbell Curl

EXERCISE INSTRUCTION

(A) Grab a barbell with an underhand grip that's about shoulder width. Let the bar hang at arm's length in front of your waist, your feet shoulder-width apart.

(B) Curl the bar up as high as you can without moving your upper arms forward.

Pause and then slowly lower the weights to the starting position.

WORKOUT C

Chin-up

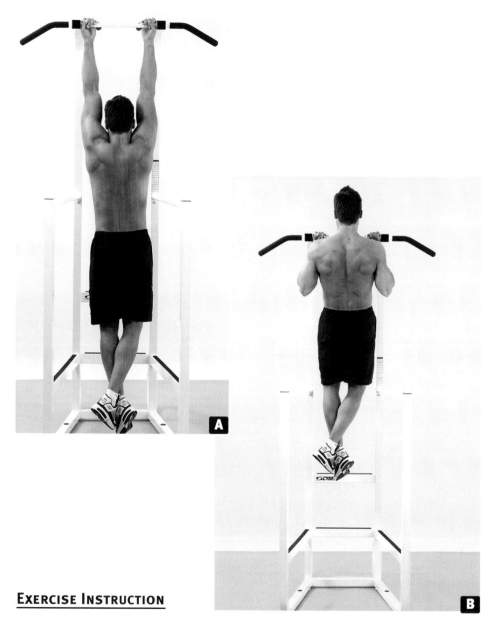

A

B

EXERCISE INSTRUCTION

(A) Grab a chin-up bar with a shoulder-width, underhand grip. Cross your ankles behind you and hang.

(B) Pull yourself up as high as you can.

Pause and then slowly return to the starting position.

Dip

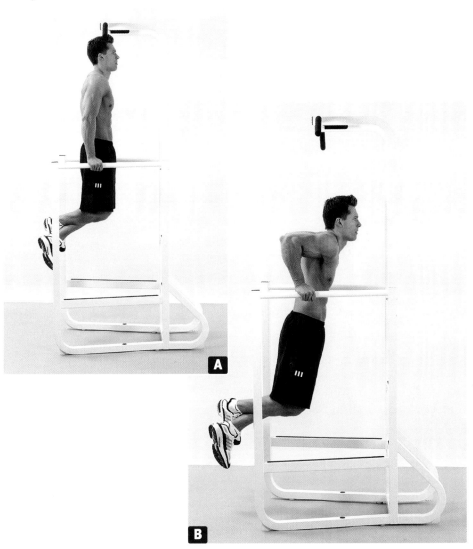

EXERCISE INSTRUCTION

(A) Grab the bars of a dip station and lift yourself so your arms are fully extended. Bend your knees and cross your ankles behind you.

(B) Bend your elbows and slowly lower your body until your upper arms are parallel to the floor.

Pause and then push yourself back up to the starting position.

CHAPTER 8 ▶

Full-Scale Fat-Loss Diet

THE FULL-SCALE FAT-LOSS DIET IS SPECIFICALLY DESIGNED to work with the Full-Scale Fat-Loss Workout on page 109. When used together, the plans will accelerate the rate at which your body sheds fat while preserving your hard-earned muscle.

You'll eat one gram of protein per pound of body weight and consume 30 percent of your total calories from fat. The remainder of your calories will come from carbohydrates. These numbers will vary by person, depending on body weight and activity level, which allows you to personalize your eating plan. To get started, follow the five-step process outlined on the next page.

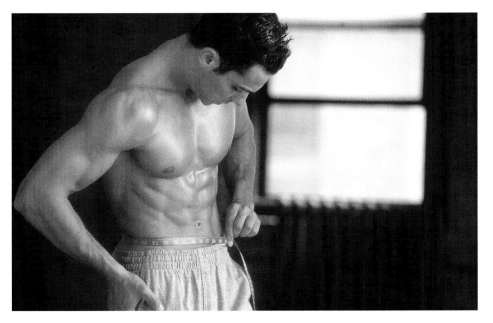

CUSTOMIZE YOUR DIET
Step 1: Calculate Your Total Calories

DAILY CALORIC EXPENDITURE FORMULA		
A. Your weight in pounds		= _____
B. Multiply A by 11 to get your resting metabolic rate	A x 11	= _____
C. Multiply B by X* to estimate your caloric expenditure through basic daily activities	B x X	= _____
D. Strength training: Multiply the number of minutes you lift weight per week by 5:	min. x 5	= _____
E. Aerobic and sprint training: Multiply the number of minutes per week that you run, cycle or play sports by 8:	min. x 8	= _____
F. Add line D and line E, and divide by 7	(D + E)/7	= _____
G. Add line C and line F to get your daily caloric needs:	C + F	= _____
H. Subtract 1000 from line G to get your daily calorie needs to lose two pounds of fat per week:	G -1000	= _____
		Total

*Determine "X" by choosing your level of daily activity, which is usually dependent on the type of workout do:
Very light (sedentary): X=1.3   Moderate (Some Activity): X=1.7
Light (Office Work): X=1.6   Heavy (Hard labor): X=2.1

Step 2: Calculate Your Protein Amount

DAILY PROTEIN FORMULA		
I. Your weight in pounds		= _____
J. Multiply A by 1 to get the total amount of protein in grams that you'll consume daily	A x 1	= _____
K. Multiply B by 4 to get the total number of calories of protein that you'll consume daily	B x 4	= _____
L. Divide C by H to get the percentage of your total calories that you'll consume from protein	C / H	= _____
		Total

Step 3: Calculate Your Fat Amount

DAILY FAT FORMULA	
M. Multiply H by 30 percent (.3) to get the total number of calories that you'll consume daily from fat	H x .3 = _____
N. Divide M by 9 to get the total amount of fat grams that you'll consume daily	M / 9 = _____ Total

Step 4: Calculate Your Carbohydrate Amount

DAILY CARBOHYDRATE FORMULA	
O. Add K and M	K + M = _____
P. Subtract O from H to get the total number of calories of carbohydrate that you'll consume daily	H - O = _____
Q. Divide P by 4 to get the total number of grams of carbohydrate that you'll consume daily	P / 4 = _____
R. Divide P by H to get the percentage of your total calories that you'll consume from carbohydrates	P / H = _____ Total

Step 5: Lose Fat

1. Eat five to six small meals a day. With the exception of your pre-and post-workout nutrition (see No. 4), try to eat both protein and fat at every meal. This will help you avoid feeling hungry and will ensure that your body has the raw materials available to make muscle. Ideally, you'll want to keep your meals relatively similar in calories. However, that's not always practical in the real world. A good rule of thumb: Eat 200 to 500 calories per meal.

2. Avoid "white" foods. You're used to avoiding these by now and it's especially important in this phase. Again, choose foods that are the lowest on the Glycemic Index (55 or lower), but cut out white bread, white rice, pasta and potatoes, including french fries, potato chips and hash browns, regardless of their GI. These aren't all "evil" but because of their low fiber content, they're not great choices.

3. Don't be afraid of fat. Remember, fat doesn't make you fat, and it makes most foods taste better. Eat healthy unsaturated fats, like olive oil, canola oil, flaxseed, peanuts, peanut butter, almonds, cashews, pine nuts and sunflower seeds. These have been shown to counteract the negative effects of saturated fats.

4. Feed your muscles. Your pre- and post-workout nutrition is extremely important. Consider it one of your meals for the day. Here's what to eat.

Pre-Workout: Consume 20 grams of protein immediately before your workout. Buy a whey protein supplement: It's ease to use and digests quickly. Of course you can eat regular food if that's more convenient. For instance, eat three ounces of tuna or about five ounces of fat-free turkey. Virtually any brand will do, but make sure that it's virtually all protein, with very little fat or carbohydrates. This will spark an increase in protein synthesis before your workout.

Post-Workout: Consume 20 grams of protein and 40 grams of carbohydrates after your workout. This will give you ample protein for

5 STEPS TO LOSE FAT FAST ►

1. Eat **5 to 6** small meals a day

2. Avoid **'white'** foods

3. Don't be afraid of **fat**

4. Feed your muscles

5. Don't obsess about the **numbers**

building muscle, as well as stimulate an increase in insulin to decrease protein breakdown. Regular food is fine, but it's probably not optimal since it's not absorbed into the bloodstream or delivered to the tissues quickly. If you crave a particular high-glycemic food (refer to www.glycemicindex.com), this is the time to eat it. In fact, the higher the better. For the best results, though, mix whey protein with maltodextrin or dextrose. They're complex carbohydrates that quickly raise blood sugar. (You can find them at any supplement store and many grocery stores.)

5. Don't obsess about the numbers. If you calculated that you should consume 38 percent of your calories from carbohydrates and you actually ate 41 percent, it's irrelevant if you were following these guidelines for fat loss, as well as the golden rules of clean eating that were discussed in Chapter 2. Likewise, if your goal was 2,200 calories and you ate 2,350, it's probably not a problem. You can balance it by eating 2,050 the next day (or simply a little less than usual), which would make your average 2,200.

SAMPLE ONE-DAY MEAL PLAN FOR A 180-POUND GUY
(approximately 2,200 calories)

Meal #1
Raisin Bran, 1.5 cups (dry)
Milk (1% fat), 1.5 cups
Orange, 1 whole
Carbohydrate: 103 g **Protein:** 22 g **Fat:** 6 g **Calories:** 554

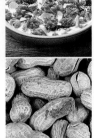

Meal #2
Peanuts, 1 oz.
Cottage cheese (2% fat), 1 cup
Carbohydrate: 14 grams **Protein:** 39 grams **Fat:** 18 grams **Calories:** 374

Meal #3
Turkey, 5 slices (or 5 oz. total weight)
Whole-grain bread, 2 slices
Mayonnaise (regular), 1 Tbsp.
Lettuce, 1 leaf
Tomato, 2 slices
Carbohydrate: 34 grams **Protein:** 34 grams **Fat:** 19 grams **Calories:** 443 grams

Meal #4
Pre-workout shake
Carbohydrate: 0 grams **Protein:** 20 grams **Fat:** 0 grams **Calories:** 80

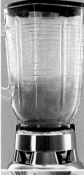

Meal #5
Post-workout shake
Carbohydrate: 40 grams **Protein:** 20 grams **Fat:** 0 grams **Calories:** 240

Meal #6
Filet mignon, 6 ounces
Steamed mixed vegetables, 1 cup
Carbohydrate: 24 grams **Protein:** 50 grams **Fat:** 28 grams **Calories:** 548

Daily totals
Calories: 2,239
Carbohydrate: 215 g; 38% of total calories
Protein: 185 g; 33% of total calories
Fat: 71g; 29% of total calories

CHAPTER 9 ▶

Instant Answers:
Full-Scale Fat-Loss Phase

THIS SUPPLEMENTAL Q AND A IS DESIGNED to answer common questions about this program, providing more details of how to execute the workouts as well as additional explanation of many of the concepts presented throughout the book.

In Stage 1, why do we do six repetitions of one workout, 20 the next and 12 the next?

Success in reducing body fat is ultimately about controlling your hormones. Insulin, cortisol, testosterone and growth hormone – to name a few – all play a role in your body composition. Eating right and getting sufficient rest and sleep will go a long way to influence your body's hormonal environment, shifting your metabolism toward fat burning rather than fat storing. But proper exercise programming can really give things a kick to accelerate the process of reducing body fat.

Training routines such as doing six repetitions of six exercises (known as the "6 + 6 method") – as you do in Workout A – have been shown to increase these key hormones to much higher levels than other methods both during and after exercise. Like a catalyst in a chemical reaction, the process of reducing body fat then becomes much easier. By utilizing 6RM weights, we also provide a stimulus that promotes retention of muscle mass. That ensures you keep all the hard-earned muscle you built in the Maximum Muscle phase – even though you're dieting.

If there's a drawback to the 6 + 6 method, it's that strength levels can be reduced for more than three days. To try to come back just a few days later and do the same workout again would be less effective because of the strength drop-off. That would quickly send you into an overtrained state with a threat of losing your hard-earned muscle. However, we can still hit the gym and be productive by shifting the training stimulus to the opposite end of the intensity spectrum. That's where the 20-rep sets come in.

Because the 20RM sets are at the far end of the intensity spectrum, they don't interfere with the recovery from the higher intensity sets from the 6 + 6 method. In fact, they can help you recover faster. The 20RM sets require lower power output and less demand on your nervous system by primarily focusing on energy systems. This is a great stimulus to increase blood flow to the working muscles to improve recovery and to raise work capacity (you remember work capacity, don't you?) for the next workout. Sort of a "use energy to get more energy" scenario.

If the 6 + 6 method is good for stimulating an optimal hormonal environment to reduce fat and hang onto your hard-earned muscle, the 12RM day comes in at a close second. On the down side, the increases in beneficial hormones are a little less than the 6 + 6 method (but still significant). On the plus side, you won't experience such a long drop-off in strength. So after a couple days of rest you're primed and ready for your next intensive day of the 6 + 6 method.

In Stage 1, why do we only do two sets of each exercise in Workout B?

Since this is primarily a "recovery" workout, there isn't a need to do a high amount of volume. Remember, this session helps you prepare for the more intense 12RM session without wearing you down.

In Stage 1, do I do an RM test like I did in the size and strength phase, or just lift?

Absolutely! The repetition maximums are specific to elicit a specific training response. Keep in mind that by the time you reach this portion of the training program, you'll be an experienced pro at determining your repetition maximums. You'll most likely hit them on your first attempt at your RM for the day.

Do the sets where I'm finding my RM for the repetition range count toward my total sets? That is, if I'm to do four sets with my 12RM (like in Workout C), do I count the first one or two sets that I use to find my 12RM?

Not unless you hit all your RMs the first time through. For instance, in Workout C, you perform the exercises as a circuit. So in the first circuit, you'll zero in on what your RM weight for each exercise is. Based on the results of that first circuit, the second circuit weights should hit the RM or be very close. That counts as your first circuit toward your total number of circuits. Same goes with each superset in Workout A and Workout B.

In Stage 1, should I use the same

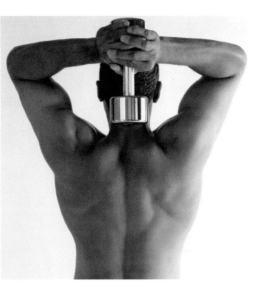

weight for each set even if I hit technical failure on an exercise before I've completed all of the prescribed number of sets?

Here's a small "tweak" for the Full-Scale Fat-Loss phase. We need to be sure that you're performing each exercise with a sufficient intensity for a specific number of sets to get the training response that we desire. Just as you have every other training day, you'll determine your repetition maximum for the day based on the training protocol. But because you'll be doing a fixed number of sets per workout, you may have to drop the weight from set to set to ensure that you complete all of the prescribed sets and reps. Therefore, if you experience a drop-off during a set – that is, you achieve technical failure – you'll simply reduce the weight by the smallest increment that will allow you to complete all the repetitions and all the sets.

Here's an example using Stage 1, Workout C: Let's say you've just completed your second set of wide-stance squats and are ready to perform your second set of 12 repetitions of dumbbell bench presses with your 12RM of 60-pound dumbbells. As you near the end of the set indicated by technical failure, you're only able to complete 10 reps. At this point, quickly reduce the weight to 55-pound dumbbells and finish the last 2 reps. When your next set of dumbbell bench presses comes around again, start with your original 12 repetition maximum of 60-pound dumbbells using the same process if necessary. So you always start with your original 12RM, but lower as necessary to complete all of the repetitions.

In Stage 2, why do we only do two exercises per workout?

Necessity. As you reach this stage of the program, you should notice that you'll need to tighten your belt a notch to keep your pants up. That's because you're losing body fat. The lower your body fat, the lower your energy reserves and your ability to recover between workouts. To load yourself with a wide variety of exercises at this point not only increases demands on training energy, but also on the energy and nutrients you need for recovery. Since you'll be three weeks into your diet, you'll have a controlled supply of nutrients from your eating plan. So you won't have as many available and risk "stealing" them from your hard-earned muscles. That will only slow progress.

Instead, we've limited the total number of exercises, but focused on the "Big Bang" exercises. These are exercises that allow us to use a lot of weight and train a lot of muscle all at once. One of the biggest mistakes guys make at during the latter durations of a fat-loss phase is to try to do too many exercises. They end up losing muscle instead of fat.

In Stage 2, why is there so much rest between exercises?

We've reduced the number of exercises to limit the draw on your energy reserves that

WHY DON'T WE DO ANY DISTANCE RUNNING FOR CARDIO?

Mainly because distance running makes you breathe hard, makes your heart race and makes you all sweaty. If you're going to do that, don't you think a woman should be involved? But seriously, it's a pretty lousy way to reduce fat and maintain muscle mass.

Here are a few reasons why:

1: Long, slow, distance running or any form of longer duration aerobic activity has been shown to interfere with strength gains. At the most basic levels, if you aren't getting stronger, you aren't gaining muscle.

2: Longer-duration aerobic activity also tends to draw energy from just about anywhere. That means it doesn't mind using some of your hard-earned muscle for energy.

3: Longer duration aerobic activity doesn't raise your resting metabolic rate, which is the number of calories you burn at rest. This program does.

4: Longer duration aerobic activity lowers your testosterone levels and increases your cortisol levels. Cortisol is a hormone that supplies the body with amino acids. Guess where it gets them? Your hard-earned muscle mass. In other words, high cortisol equals a loss of muscle. Just as important, testosterone is the hormone that gives you hair in funny places, makes you want to jump your significant other and is necessary to build muscle. Need more explanation?

5: Longer duration aerobic activity may be the most boring activity on the planet.

If you need a real-world example to see the differences between longer duration aerobic activity and the form of energy system training recommended in this program, just look at the sprinters compared to the marathoners in the Olympics. Sprinters run repeated intervals of short distances and look lean and muscular. Marathoners run long distances for long periods of time and look like they went on a hunger strike. Enough said.

you'll use to train your muscles and to recover. However, you also need sufficient total sets to keep all the muscle you gained. If we cut rest periods too short, the amount of weight you'll be able to use at this stage wouldn't keep muscle on your grandma.

By resting sufficiently, you can keep your training intensity very high and extend the number of sets per exercise. This assures sufficient stimulus to keep all the muscle that you've gained. In other words, slap some weight on the bar and train it into the ground!

In Stage 2, do I do an RM test like I did in the size and strength phase, or just lift?

Has there been any guesswork in the program so far? Of course not and we're not about to start now. Just as we have at each stage of this training program, we want to assure that training intensity is optimal. Because energy is a little more variable at this stage of the program, we've provided you a range rather than a specific repetition maximum. Use the first weight you hit that allows you to train in that repetition range (four to six) and stick with it for as many sets as your mental intensity and energy reserves allow you to avoid technical failure.

Why do we only do one ab exercise in this entire phase?

We think you miscounted. A quick look at the whole phase shows about 17 different exercises that will influence the abdominal region.

What a lot of guys don't understand is that any exercise performed in the standing position or that requires a fixed or stabilized spinal position requires a great deal of abdominal activity and strength. It's not just about the amount of direct work you do for your abdominal muscles but also how much indirect work you do.

Developing a good looking "six-pack" requires that you uncover the abdominal muscles by stripping away the fat and has very little to do with which abdominal exercises you do.

In fact, it could be argued that you may never have to do any direct abdominal exercises to develop enviable abs.

How do I know if I'm eating too much?

You won't be losing weight. Just like in the Maximum Muscle phase, you should check your weight weekly on a scale. The day you start the plan, weigh yourself in the morning, after you've gone to the restroom, but before you eat breakfast. The following week, weigh yourself again, following the same procedure. If you have a "sizable" amount of fat to lose – you're 20 pounds overweight, for instance – you should be losing at the rate of about two pounds a week. If you're losing less, drop your calories by 250 per day. Then continue this process each week until you're losing around two pounds a week. You can lose faster, but cap your losses at three pounds per week. That's because more than that and you're really putting your hard-earned muscle at risk. Also, regardless of your rate of fat loss, keep your calories around 2,000 per day. Eat significantly fewer calories – say, 300 or more – and you risk lowering your metabolism and using your muscle for energy. That not only slows the rate at which your body burns fat, it'll make you look and feel weak and flabby. (Think of it as "skinny-fat.")

If you're fairly lean already, don't concern yourself much with the scale-weight, except to make sure that you're not losing too much, too fast. You should visibly notice that you're losing fat and your clothes should start fitting better.

Either way, don't obsess too much about calories. Simply eat the foods that we've recommended and always follow the pre- and post-workout nutrition recommendations. Then simply monitor your progress and eat a little less or a little more until you're getting the desired results.

PART IV

THE
FINAL
DETAILS

CHAPTER 10 ▶

Bonus Phase:
Chest and Arms Specialization

THIS IS A FOUR-WEEK CYCLE THAT'S DESIGNED TO MAXIMIZE YOUR CHEST AND ARM SIZE, while maintaining the gains you've made in your other body parts throughout this program. It includes two parts: weight training and energy system training. Follow the directions given for each.

THE WEIGHT WORKOUT
STAGE 1: WEEKS 1 to 2

Warm-up: Before each workout, do two to three circuits of either Warm-up No. 1 or Warm-up No. 2 (your choice). (Perform your ramp-up warm-up as described in Chapter 1 prior to the appropriate exercises.)

Frequency: Perform each workout once a week, resting at least a day between each. So you might do Workout A on Monday, Workout B on Wednesday and Workout C on Friday.

Exercise order: Perform the exercises using either straight sets or alternating sets. Straight sets will be designated simply as a number – for instance, 2 or 5. Alternating sets will be designated as a number and letter pair – for instance, 1A and 1B or 2A, 2B and 2C. For straight sets, complete all sets of that exercise – resting between each set – before moving on to the next. For alternating sets, perform the exercises as a modified circuit. That is, do one set of each exercise after the other, but rest in between each. If the alternating set consists of two exercises (1A and 1B, for instance), you'll perform one set of the first exercise, rest, then do one set of the second exercise and rest again, alternating back and forth until you've completed all sets of both exercises. If the alternating set consists of three exercises (2A, 2B and 2C, for instance), you'll perform one set of the first exercise, rest, do one set of the second exercise, rest and then do one set of the third exercise and rest again, alternating back and forth until you've completed all sets of all three exercises.

Rest: Between sets and exercises, rest only as long as it takes for your breathing rate to approach normal. This time period should never exceed two minutes.

Repetitions and weights

These workouts are a little more varied and use a few more tricks than the ones that you've performed elsewhere in the book. So we'll explain the specifics of how to do each exercise in greater detail than usual.

Workout A

1A: Isometric Bench Press

Week 1: Hold for 40 seconds in the "pause" position (see exercise description). If you can't hold the weight for at least 38 to 40 seconds, the weight is too heavy; if you can hold it for longer than 42 seconds, it's too light. (In other words, allow yourself a couple of seconds in either direction.) After you've found the right weight, do as many sets as you can until you can't hold the weight for 40 seconds.

Week 2: Perform the exercise the same way, but hold in the pause position for 30 seconds.

1B: External Rotation

Weeks 1 and 2: Do as many sets of eight repetitions with your 8RM weight as you can. When you drop-off (achieve technical failure), you've completed the exercise for the day.

1C. Incline Fly to Press

Week 1: Use your 10RM weight for the incline fly and perform sets until you can't do at least eight repetitions without achieving technical failure. (So you'll lift in the 8 to 10 repetition range, ending each set when you achieve technical failure.) Take five seconds to lower the weight each repetition; that means you'll probably have to use a lighter weight than if you were lifting faster. As soon as you reach your drop-off, perform the incline press to technical failure (see exercise description).

Week 2: Perform the exercise the same way,

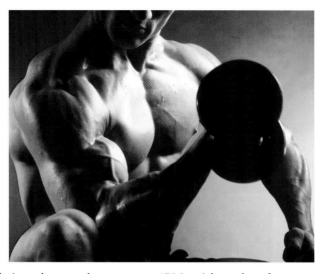

but use your 8RM weight and perform sets until you can't do at least six repetitions without achieving technical failure.

2A. Three-Stop Decline Dumbbell Triceps Extension

Weeks 1 and 2: Do as many sets as you can with a weight that allows you to hold for 10 seconds in the second "stop" position (see exercise description). As a general rule, if you can't hold the position for longer than eight seconds, the weight is too heavy; if you can hold it for more than 12 seconds, it's too light.

2B. Incline Hammer Curl

Weeks 1 and 2: Use your 8RM weight and perform sets until you can't do at least six repetitions without achieving technical failure. (So you'll work out in the six- to eight-repetition range, ending each set when you achieve technical failure.) Take five seconds to lower the weight each repetition; that means you'll probably have to use a lighter weight than if you were lifting faster.

Workout B

1. Squat

Week 1: Use your 10RM weight and perform sets until you can't do at least eight repetitions without achieving technical failure. (So you'll work out in the eight- to 10-repetition range, ending each set when you achieve technical failure.)

Week 2: Use your 8RM weight and perform sets until you can't do at least six repetitions without achieving technical failure. (So you'll work out in the six- to eight-repetition range, ending each set when you achieve technical failure.)

2. Close-Grip Chin-up

Weeks 1 and 2: Do as many repetitions as possible (AMRAP), stopping the set when you achieve technical failure. Simply match the number of sets you do with the number that you were able to do in the previous exercise (squat).

3. Lean-Away Lateral Raise

Weeks 1 and 2: Use your 20RM weight and perform sets until you can't do at least 12 repetitions without achieving technical failure. (So you'll work out in the 12- to 20-repetition range, ending each set when you achieve technical failure.)

4. Hanging Leg Raise

Weeks 1 and 2: Do as many repetitions as possible (AMRAP), stopping the set when you achieve technical failure. Simply match the number of sets you do with the number that you were able to do in the previous exercise (lean-away lateral raise).

Workout C
1A. Incline Dumbbell Press with Pause

Week 1: Use your 8RM weight and perform sets until you can't do at least six repetitions without achieving technical failure. (So you'll workout out in the six- to eight-repetition range, ending each set when you achieve technical failure.) At the bottom – or stretch position – of the lift, pause for four seconds before pressing the weight back up. That means you'll

probably have to use a lighter weight than you would for your normal 8RM.

Week 2: Use your 6RM weight and perform sets until you can't do at least four repetitions without achieving technical failure. (So you'll work out in the four- to six-repetition range, ending each set when you achieve technical failure.) At the bottom – or stretch position – of the lift, pause for four seconds before pressing the weight back up. That means you'll probably have to use a lighter weight than you would for your normal 6RM.

1B. Incline Lower Trap Raise

Weeks 1 and 2: Do as many sets of 10 repetitions with your 10RM weight as you can. When you drop-off (achieve technical failure), you've completed the exercise for the day.

1C. Dumbbell Bench Press

Week 1: Use your 20RM weight and perform sets until you can't do at least 12 repetitions without achieving technical failure. (So you'll work out in the 12- to 20-repetition range, ending each set when you achieve technical failure.)

Week 2: Use your 15RM weight and perform sets until you can't do at least nine repetitions without achieving technical failure. (So you'll work out in the nine- to 15-repetition range, ending each set when you achieve technical failure.)

2A. Telle Curl

Weeks 1 and 2: Do as many sets of six repetitions with your 6RM weight as you can. When you drop-off (achieve technical failure), you've completed the exercise for the day.

2B. Incline Barbell Triceps Extension

Weeks 1 and 2: Do as many sets of eight repetitions with your 8RM as you can. When you drop-off (achieve technical failure), you've completed the exercise for the day.

Take five seconds to lower the weight each repetition; that means you'll probably have to use a lighter weight than if you were lifting faster.

ENERGY SYSTEM TRAINING
STAGE 1: WEEKS 1 to 2
HOW TO DO IT

Do Energy System Training (EST) A on the day following Weight Workout A. Do EST B on the day following Weight Workout B. So you'll perform EST A on Tuesday and EST B on Thursday.

EST A

Week 1: Do six 15-second sprints at 100 per-cent of your full effort, resting for 60 seconds between each.

Week 2: Do eight 15-second sprints at 100 percent of your full effort, resting for 60 seconds between each.

EST B

Week 1: Do five 30-second sprints at 100 per-cent of your full effort, resting for 120 seconds between each.

Week 2: Do six 30-second sprints at 100 per-cent of your full effort, resting for 120 seconds between each.

AT A GLANCE: CHEST & ARMS SPECIALIZATION WORKOUT (STAGE 1)

	Monday	Tuesday	Wednesday	Thursday	Friday	Saturday	Sunday
Week 1	WW A	EST A	WW B	EST B	WW C	rest	rest
Week 2	WW A	EST A	WW B	EST B	WW C	rest	rest

AT A GLANCE: WORKOUT A (STAGE 1)

EXERCISE	INTENSITY	SETS	REPS
Warmup #1 or #2	Bar	2-3	5
1A. Isometric Bench Press			
Week 1	40S-RM	N	1
Week 2	30S-RM	N	1
1B. External Rotation			
Week 1	8RM	N	8
Week 2	8RM	N	8
1C. Incline Fly to Press			
Week 1 (Incline Fly)	10RM	N	8-10
Week 1 (Incline Press)	Fly Weight	1	AMRAP
Week 2 (Incline Fly)	8RM	N	6-8
Week 2 (Incline Press)	Fly Weight	1	AMRAP
2A. Three-Stop Decline Dumbbell Triceps Extension			
Week 1	3-Stop-RM	N	1
Week 2	3-Stop-RM	N	1
2B. Incline Hammer Curl			
Week 1	8RM	N	6-8
Week 2	8RM	N	6-8
Week 3	6RM	3	6

*N = the number of sets it takes you to reach technical failure

AT A GLANCE: WORKOUT B (STAGE 1)

EXERCISE	INTENSITY	SETS	REPS
Warmup #1 or #2 Bar		2-3	5
1. Squat			
Week 1	10RM	N	8-10
Week 2	8RM	N	6-8
2. Close-Grip Chin-up			
Week 1	Body	N	AMRAP
Week 2	Body	N	AMRAP
3. Lean-Away Lateral Raise			
Week 1	20RM	N	12-20
Week 2	20RM	N	12-20
4. Hanging Leg Raise			
Week 1	Body	N	AMRAP
Week 2	Body	N	AMRAP

*N = the number of sets it takes you to reach technical failure

AT A GLANCE: WORKOUT C (STAGE 1)

EXERCISE	INTENSITY	SETS	REPS
Warmup #1 or #2 Bar		2-3	5
1A. Incline Dumbbell Bench Press with Pause			
Week 1	8RM	N	6-8
Week 2	6RM	N	4-6
1B. Incline Lower Trap Raise			
Week 1	10RM	N	10
Week 2	10RM	N	10
1C. Dumbbell Bench Press			
Week 1	20RM	N	12-20
Week 2	15RM	N	9-15
2A. Telle Curl			
Week 1	6RM	N	6
Week 2	6RM	N	6
2B. Incline Barbell Triceps Extension			
Week 1	8RM	N	8
Week 2	8RM	N	8

*N = the number of sets it takes you to reach technical failure

WORKOUT A

Isometric Bench Press

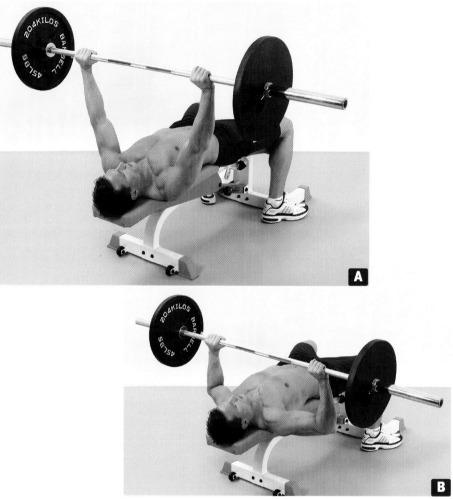

EXERCISE INSTRUCTION

(A) Lie on your back on a flat bench with your feet flat on the floor. Your lower back should be in a naturally arched position – don't flatten it or try to arch to a greater extent at any time during the lift. Grip the bar with your hands just wider than shoulder-width apart and lift the bar off the uprights.

(B) Lower the bar until it's about four inches off your chest or until your upper arms are parallel to the floor.

Hold that position for 40 seconds to complete one set.

Caution: Always use a spotter or perform this exercise in a squat rack with the safety bars set just above chest level.

External Rotation

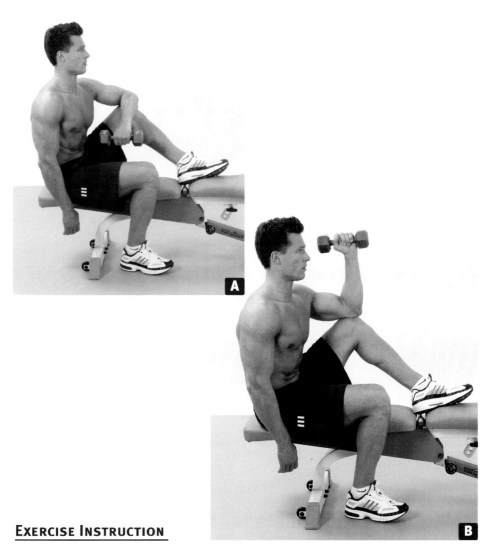

EXERCISE INSTRUCTION

(A) Grab a dumbbell in your left hand and sit on a bench. Place your left foot flat on the bench with your knee bent.

(B) Bend your left elbow 90 degrees and place it on your left knee.

Without changing the bend in your elbow, rotate your upper arm up and back as far as you can. (Your forearm will swing like a gate on hinges.)

Pause, then return to the starting position.

WORKOUT A

Incline Fly to Press

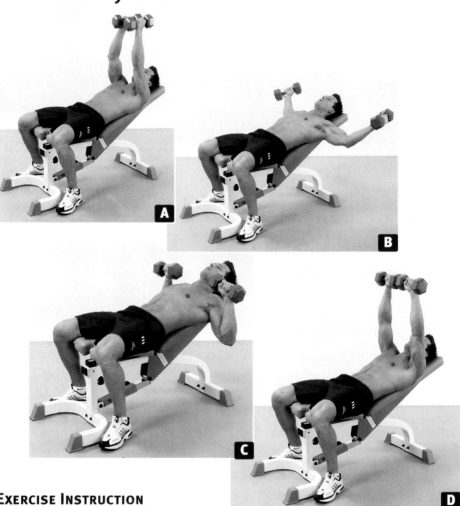

EXERCISE INSTRUCTION

(A) Grab a pair of dumbbells and lie on your back on a bench set to a low incline (about 15 degrees). Lift the dumbbells so they're over your chin and hold them over your chest with your elbows slightly bent and your palms facing each other.

(B) Slowly lower the dumbbells down and slightly back until your upper arms are parallel to the floor and in line with your ears.

Pause, then lift the dumbbells back to the starting position.

Once you achieve technical failure, complete as many dumbbell bench presses as you can by bending your elbows and lowering the weight to the sides of your chest (C), then pushing the dumbbells up and together (D).

When you achieve technical failure on the dumbbell bench press, move on to the next exercise.

Three-Stop Decline Dumbbell Triceps Extension

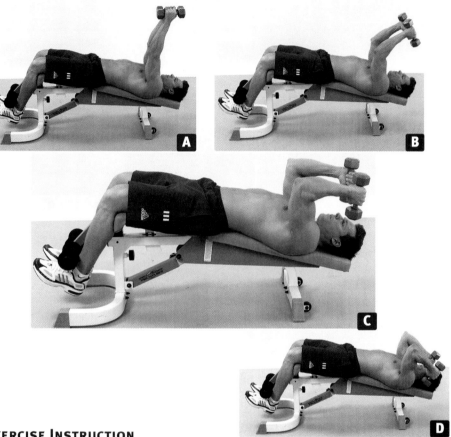

EXERCISE INSTRUCTION

(A) Grab a pair of dumbbells and lie on your back on a decline bench, your feet securely hooked under the supports. Hold the dumbbells over your chin at arm's length, your palms facing each other.

(B) Without moving your upper arms, lower the weights a few inches and pause for 10 seconds (first stop).

(C) Lower the weight until your elbows are bent 90 degrees and pause for 10 seconds (second stop).

(D) Lower the weight a few more inches (your lower arms will be below parallel to the floor) and pause for 10 seconds (third stop). That's one set.

When you can't hold the second stop for 10 seconds, move on to the next exercise.

Pause, then raise the dumbbells back to the starting position by straightening your arms.

WORKOUT A
Incline Hammer Curl

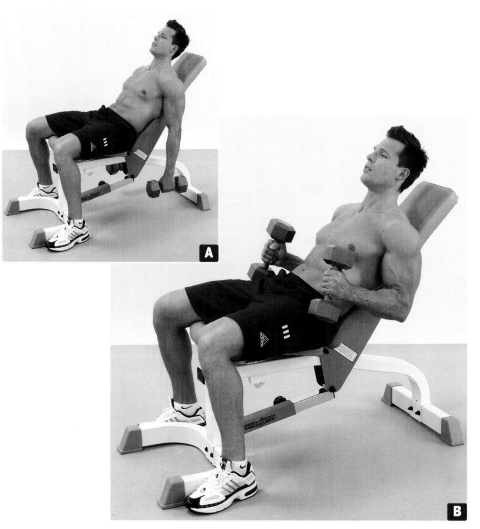

EXERCISE INSTRUCTION

(A) Set an incline bench to a 45-degree angle. Grab a pair of dumbbells and lie on your back on the bench. Let your arms hang straight down from your shoulders, your palms facing each other.

(B) Without allowing your upper arm to move forward, slowly curl the weights up as high as you can.

Pause, then take a full five seconds to lower the dumbbells back to the starting position.

Squat

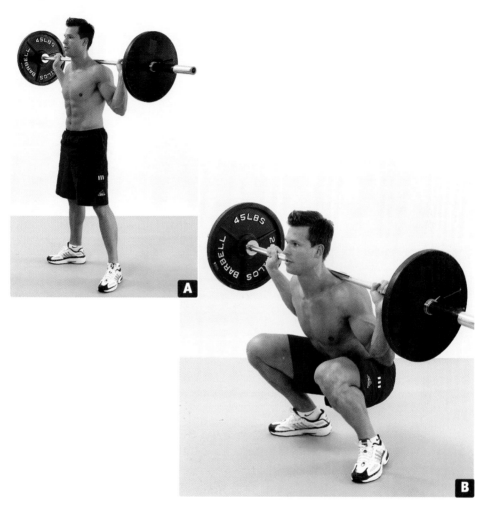

EXERCISE INSTRUCTION

(A) Hold a bar across your upper back with an overhand grip, your feet set shoulder-width apart and your shoulders pulled back.

(B) Slowly lower your body as far as possible – or until your thighs are at least parallel to the floor – keeping your back naturally arched and your lower legs nearly perpendicular to the floor.

Pause and then return to the starting position.

WORKOUT B

Close-Grip Chin-up

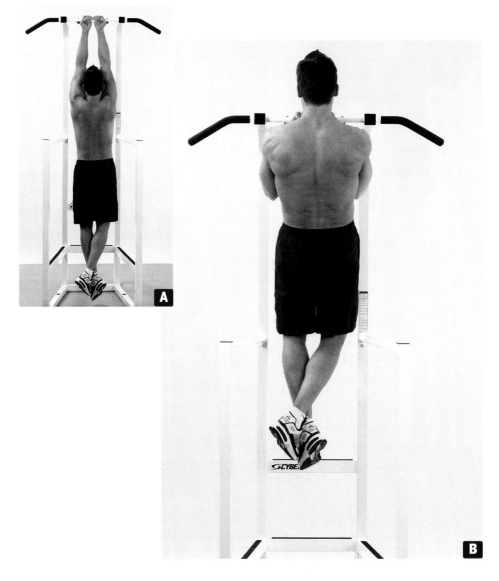

EXERCISE INSTRUCTION

(A) Grab the chin-up bar with an underhand grip, your hands about six to eight inches apart, and hang with your ankles crossed behind you.

(B) Pull yourself up as high as you can.

Pause, then slowly return to the starting position.

Lean-Away Lateral Raise

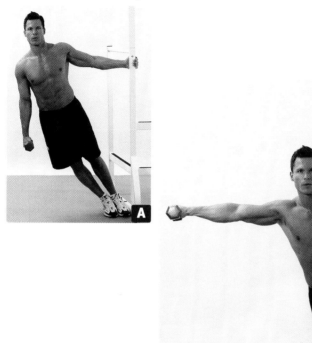

EXERCISE INSTRUCTION

(A) Hold a dumbbell in your right hand at arm's length next to your side and stand with your left leg next to a sturdy object, such as a power rack. Place your right foot next to your right, grab the power rack with your left hand and allow your left arm to straighten so that you're leaning significantly to your right. (Your body, arms and legs will form a triangle with the power rack.) The palm of your right hand should be facing your body and your right elbow should be bent slightly.

(B) Without changing the bend in your elbow, raise your right arm until it's parallel to the floor.

Pause, then return to the starting position.

Once you've performed all of the prescribed repetitions, turn around and perform the same movement with your left arm.

WORKOUT B
Hanging Leg Raise

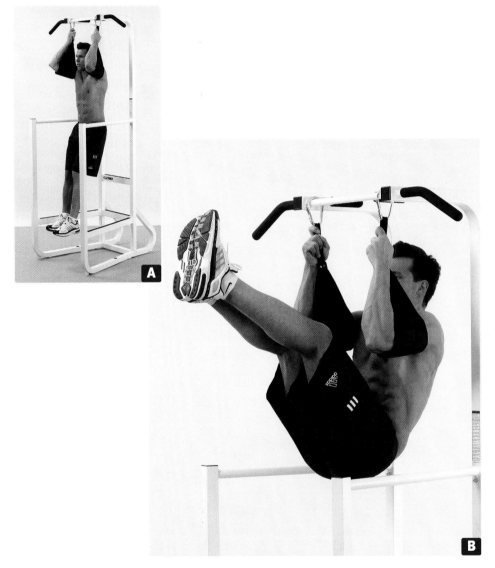

EXERCISE INSTRUCTION

(A) Grab a chin-up bar with an overhand, shoulder-width grip and hang from the bar with your knees slightly bent and feet together. (Use elbow supports if they're available.)

(B) Pull your hips up and in, lifting your knees as close to your chest as possible. Pause, then slowly lower your legs to the starting position.

Incline Dumbbell Press with Pause

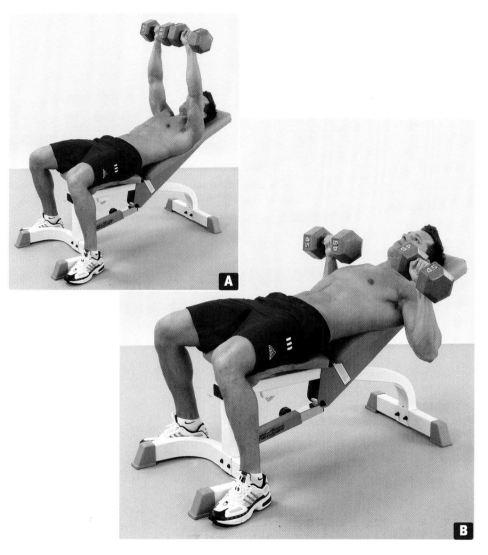

EXERCISE INSTRUCTION

(A) Grab a pair of dumbbells and lie on your back on a bench set to a low incline (15 to 30 degrees). Lift the dumbbells up at arm's length so they're over your chin and hold them with your palms turned toward your feet so that your thumbs are facing each other.

(B) Slowly lower the weights to your upper chest.

Pause for a full four seconds, then push them back up over your chin.

WORKOUT C
Incline Lower Trap Raise

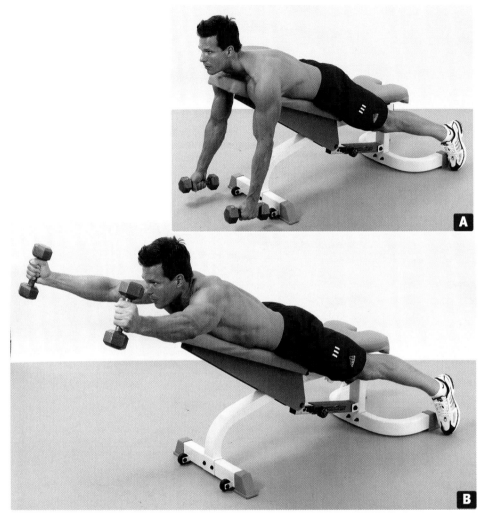

EXERCISE INSTRUCTION

(A) Set an incline bench to a 30-degree angle. Grab a pair of dumbbells and lie with your chest against the pad. Let your arms hang straight down from your shoulders and turn your palms so they're facing each other. Keep your elbows slightly bent.

(B) Without changing the bend in your elbows, raise your arms at a 45-degree angle to your body (so that they form a "Y") until they're in line with your torso.

Pause, then slowly lower the weights to the starting position.

Dumbbell Bench Press

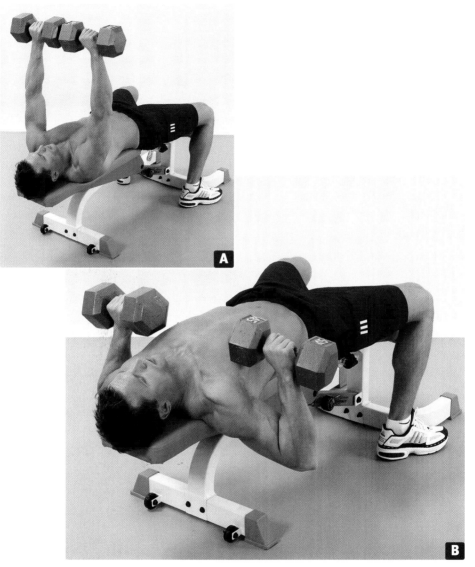

EXERCISE INSTRUCTION

(A) Grab a pair of dumbbells and lie on your back on a flat bench, holding the dumbbells over your chest.

(B) Lower the dumbbells to the sides of your chest, pause, then push them back up to the starting position.

WORKOUT C

Telle Curl

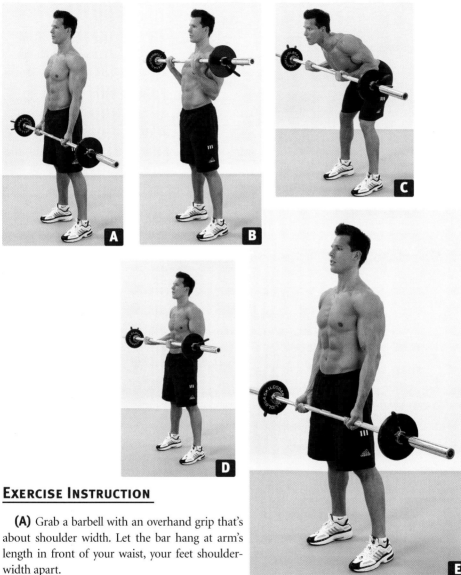

EXERCISE INSTRUCTION

(A) Grab a barbell with an overhand grip that's about shoulder width. Let the bar hang at arm's length in front of your waist, your feet shoulder-width apart.

(B) Curl the bar up as high as you can without moving your upper arms forward and hold it in that position.

(C) Keeping your back naturally arched, bend forward at the hips until your forearms are parallel to the floor.

(D) Pause, then raise your torso back to an upright position while keeping your fore-arms parallel to the floor. (Your arms will straighten slightly.)

(E) Lower the weights back to the starting position and repeat.

Incline Barbell Triceps Extension

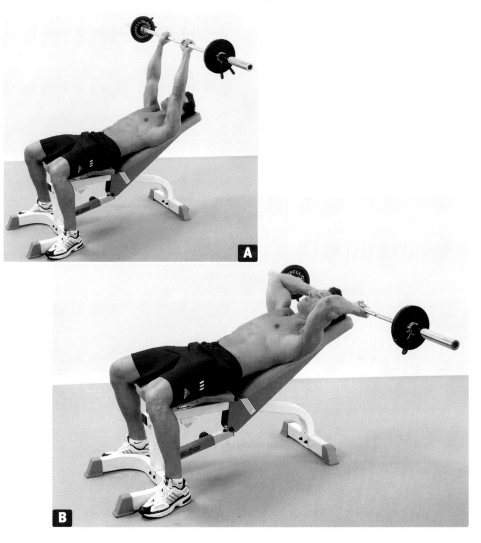

EXERCISE INSTRUCTION

(A) Lie on your back on an incline bench set to a 30-degree angle. Hold a barbell above your chin with an overhand grip, your hands about shoulder-width apart.

(B) Without moving your upper arms, take a full five seconds to lower the bar until your lower arms are beyond parallel to the floor.

Pause, then raise the bar back to the starting position by straightening your arms.

THE WEIGHT WORKOUT
STAGE 2: WEEKS 3 to 4
HOW TO DO IT

Warm-up: Before each workout, do two to three circuits of either Warm-up No. 1 or Warm-up No. 2 (your choice). (Perform your ramp-up warm-up as described in Chapter 1 for prior to the appropriate exercises.)

Frequency: Perform each workout once a week, resting at least a day between each. So you might do Workout A on Monday, Workout B on Wednesday and Workout C on Friday.

Exercise Order: Perform the exercises using either straight sets or alternating sets. Straight sets will be designated simply as a number – for instance, "2" or "5." Alternating sets will be designated as a number and letter pair – for instance, "1A" and "1B" or "2A", "2B" and "2C." For straight sets, complete all sets of that exercise – resting between each set – before moving on to the next. For alternating sets, perform the exercises as a modified circuit. That is, do one set of each exercise after the other, but rest in between each. If the alternating set consists of two exercises (1A and 1B, for instance), you'll perform one set of the first exercise, rest, then do one set of the second exercise and rest again, alternating back and forth until you've completed all sets of both exercises. If the alternating set consists of three exercises (2A, 2B and 2C, for instance), you'll perform one set of the first exercise, rest, do one set of the second exercise, rest and then do one set of the third exercise and rest again, alternating back and forth until you've completed all sets of all three exercises.

Rest: Between sets and exercises, rest only as long as it takes for your breathing rate to approach normal. This time period should never exceed two minutes.

REPETITIONS AND WEIGHTS

These workouts are a little more varied and use a few more tricks than the ones that you've performed elsewhere in the book. So we'll explain the specifics of how to do each exercise in greater detail than usual.

Workout A:
1. Bench Press
Weeks 3 and 4:

Set 1: Do one set of six repetitions with your 6RM. Rest.

Sets 2 to N: Drop the initial weight by 15 percent and do as many sets of six repetitions as possible. When you can only complete five repetitions (without achieving technical failure), immediately and without resting do your final set (below).

Final Set: Use a weight that's 40 percent of the weight you used in your first set and do as many repetitions as possible, stopping when you achieve technical failure.

2A. Static Curl
Week 3: Hold for 40 seconds in the "pause" position (see exercise description). If you can't hold the weight for at least 38 to 40 seconds, the weight is too heavy; if you can hold it for longer than 42 seconds, it's too light. (In other words, allow yourself a couple of seconds in either direction.) After you've found the right weight, do as many sets as you can until you can't hold the weight for 40 seconds.

Week 4: Perform the same way, but hold for 30 seconds.

2B. Static Lying Triceps Extension
Week 3: Hold for 40 seconds in the "pause" position (see exercise description). If you can't hold the weight for at least 38 to 40 seconds, the weight is too heavy; if you can hold it for longer than 42 seconds, it's too light. (In other words, allow yourself a couple of seconds in either direction.) After you've found the right weight, do as many sets as you can until you can't hold the weight for 40 seconds.

Week 4: Perform the same way, but hold for 30 seconds.

Workout B

1. Neutral-Grip Chin-up

Week 3: Do three sets, performing as many repetitions as possible (AMRAP) each time, stopping the set when you achieve technical failure.

Week 4: Do as many sets of five repetitions with your 5RM weight as you can. When you drop-off (achieve technical failure), you've completed the exercise for the day. (You may need to hang a dipping belt around your weight to increase the load.)

2. Sidelying Lateral Raise

Weeks 3 and 4: Use your 20RM weight and perform sets until you can't do at least 12 repetitions without achieving technical failure. (So you'll work out in the 12- to 20- repetition range, ending each set when you achieve technical failure.)

3. Snatch-Grip Deadlift on Box

Week 3: Use your 8RM weight and do three sets of six to eight repetitions.

Week 4: Use your 6RM weight and do three sets of four to six repetitions.

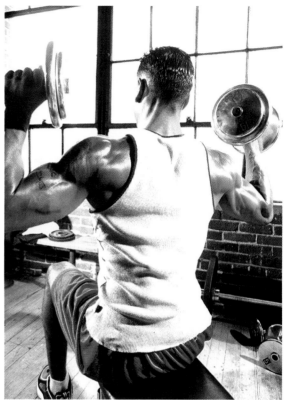

Workout C

1A. Incline Dip

Week 3: Do as many sets of eight repetitions with your 8RM weight as you can. When you drop-off (achieve technical failure), you've completed the exercise for the day. (You may need to hang a dipping belt around your weight to increase the load.)

Week 4: Do as many sets of six repetitions with your 6RM weight as you can. When you drop-off (achieve technical failure), you've completed the exercise for the day. (You may need to hang a dipping belt around your weight to increase the load.)

1B. Incline Dumbbell Press

Week 3: Use your 20RM weight and perform sets until you can't do at least 12 repetitions without achieving technical failure. (So you'll work out in the 12 to 20 repetition range, ending each set when you achieve technical failure.)

Week 4: Use your 15RM weight and perform sets until you can't do at least nine repetitions without achieving technical failure. (So you'll work out in the nine- to 15-repetition range, ending each set when you achieve technical failure.)

2A. Swiss-ball Lying to Sitting Offset Dumbbell Curl

Week 3: Do as many sets of 12 repetitions with your 12RM weight as you can. When you drop-off (achieve technical failure), you've completed the exercise for the day.

Week 4: Do as many sets of eight repetitions with your 8RM weight as you can. When you drop-off (achieve technical failure), you've completed the exercise for the day.

2B. Lying Triceps Extension to Close-Grip Bench Press

Week 3: Do as many sets of 12 repetitions with your 12RM weight as you can. As soon as you drop-off (achieve technical failure), without resting perform the incline press to technical failure (see exercise description).

Week 4: Perform the same way, but do as many sets of eight repetitions with your 8RM weight as you can.

ENERGY SYSTEM TRAINING
STAGE 2: WEEKS 3-4
HOW TO DO IT

Do Energy System Training (EST) A on the day following Weight Workout A. Do EST B on the day following Weight Workout B. So you'll perform EST A on Tuesday and EST B on Thursday.

EST A

Week 3: Do 10 15-second sprints at 100 percent of your full effort, resting for 60 seconds between each.

Week 4: Do 12 15-second sprints at 100 percent of your full effort, resting for 60 seconds between each.

EST B

Week 3: Do seven 30-second sprints at 100 percent of your full effort, resting for 120 seconds between each.

Week 4: Do eight 30-second sprints at 100 percent of your full effort, resting for 120 seconds between each.

AT A GLANCE: CHEST & ARMS SPECIALIZATION WORKOUT (STAGE 2)

	Monday	Tuesday	Wednesday	Thursday	Friday	Saturday	Sunday
Week 1	WW A	EST A	WW B	EST B	WW C	rest	rest
Week 2	WW A	EST A	WW B	EST B	WW C	rest	rest

AT A GLANCE: WORKOUT A (STAGE 2)

	EXERCISE	INTENSITY	SETS	REPS
Warmup #1 or #2		Bar	2-3	5
1A. Bench Press				
Week 1	Set 1	6RM	1	6
	Set 2	6RM-15%	N	6
	Final Set	6RM-40%	1	AMRAP
Week 2	Set 1	6RM	1	6
	Set 2	6RM-15%	N	6
	Final Set	6RM-40%	1	AMRAP
1B. Static Curl				
Week 1		40S-RM	N	1
Week 2		30S-RM	N	1
1C. Static Lying Triceps Extension				
Week 1		40S-RM	N	1
Week 2		30S-RM	N	1

*N = the number of sets it takes you to reach technical failure

AT A GLANCE: WORKOUT B (Stage 2)

EXERCISE	INTENSITY	SETS	REPS
Warmup #1 or #2 Bar		2-3	5
1. Neutral-Grip Chin-up			
Week 1	Body	3	AMRAP
Week 2	5RM	N	5
2. Sidelying Lateral Raise			
Week 1	20RM	N	12-20
Week 2	20RM	N	12-20
3. Snatch-Grip Deadlift on Box			
Week 1	8RM	3	6-8
Week 2	6RM	3	4-6

*N = the number of sets it takes you to reach technical failure

AT A GLANCE: WORKOUT C (Stage 2)

EXERCISE	INTENSITY	SETS	REPS
Warmup #1 or #2	Bar	2-3	5
1A. Incline Dip			
Week 3	8RM	N	8
Week 4	6RM	N	6
2B. Incline Dumbbell Press			
Week 3	20RM	N	12-20
Week 4	15RM	N	9-15
2A. Swiss-ball Lying to Sitting Offset Dumbbell Curl			
Week 3	12RM	N	12
Week 4	8RM	N	8
2B. Lying Triceps Extension to Close-Grip Bench Press			
Week 3 (Lying Triceps Extension)	12RM	N	12
Week 3 (Close-Grip Bench Press)	Ext. Weight	1	AMRAP
Week 4 (Lying Triceps Extension)	8RM	N	8
Week 4 (Close-Grip Bench Press)	Ext. Weight	1	AMRAP

*N = the number of sets it takes you to reach technical failure

WORKOUT A

Bench Press

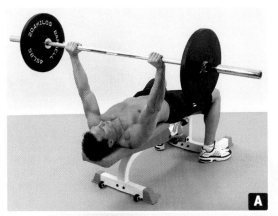

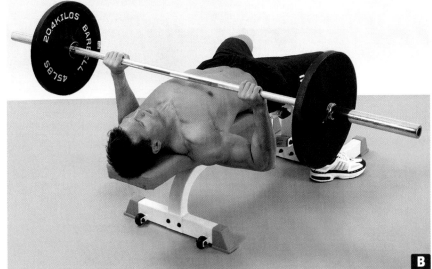

EXERCISE INSTRUCTION

(A) Lie on your back on a flat bench with your feet flat on the floor. Your lower back should be in a naturally arched position – don't flatten it or try to arch to a greater extent at any time during the lift. Grab the bar with your hands just wider than shoulder-width apart. Lift the bar off the uprights and hold it over your chest at arm's length.

(B) Lower the bar to your chest, keeping your elbows pulled close to your sides (your upper arms will be at about a 45-degree angle to your body in the "down" position).

Pause, then push the bar back to the starting position.

Static Curl

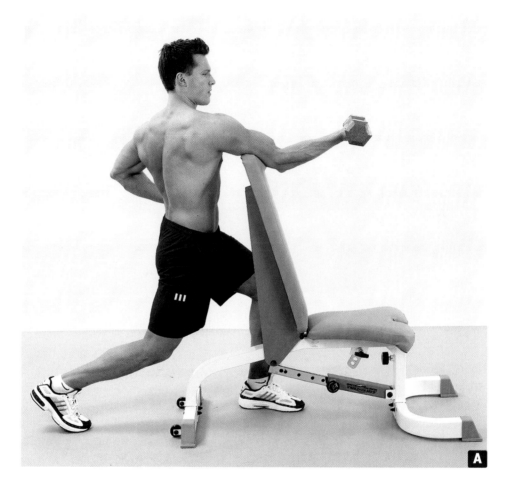

EXERCISE INSTRUCTION

(A) Grab a dumbbell with your right hand and stand behind a raised incline bench. Place the back of your upper arm across the top of the bench so that only the mid-part of your arm is touching it. Lower the dumbbell until your arm is bent about 20 degrees.

Hold that position for 40 seconds. Repeat with your right arm. That's one set.

WORKOUT A

Static Lying Triceps Extension

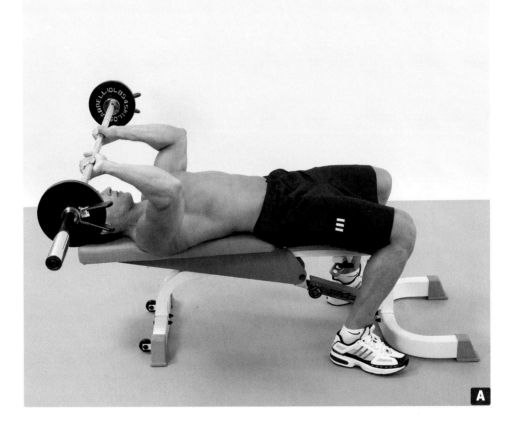

EXERCISE INSTRUCTION

(A) Grab a barbell and lie on your back on a flat bench. Hold the barbell straight above your shoulders in an overhand grip, your hands about shoulder-width apart. Without moving your upper arms, lower the bar until your elbows are bent 90 degrees.

Hold that position for 40 seconds. That's one set.

WORKOUT B

Neutral-Grip Chin-up

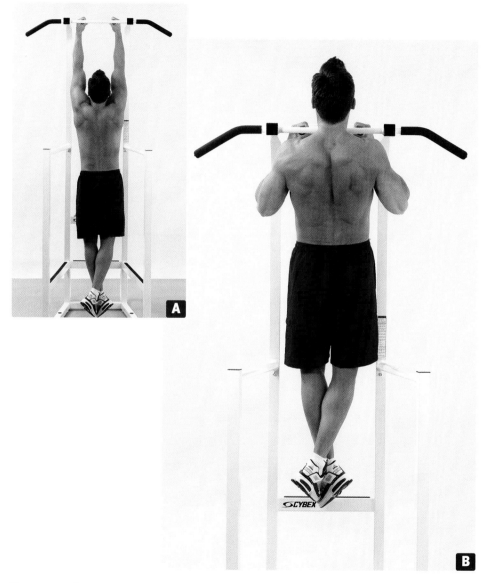

Exercise Instruction

(A) Hang from the parallel chin-up bars using an overhand grip with your palms facing each other. Cross your feet behind you.

(B) Pull yourself up until your chest is as close to your hands as possible. Pause, then slowly lower yourself to the starting position.

WORKOUT B
Sidelying Lateral Raise

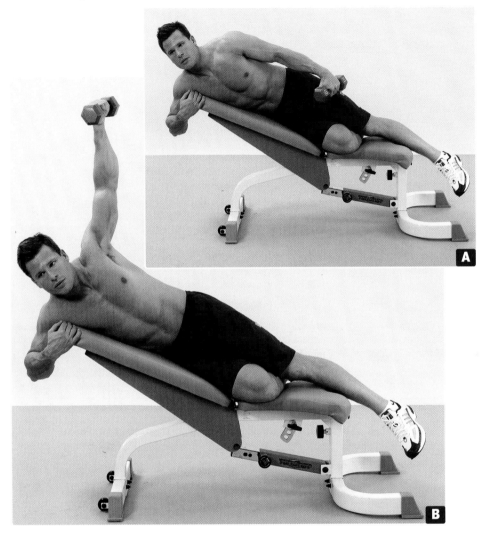

EXERCISE INSTRUCTION

(A) Grab a dumbbell in your left hand and lie on your right side on an incline bench set that's set to 15 degrees. Hold the dumbbell next to your left side with your elbow slightly bent.

(B) Without changing the bend in your elbow, raise your arm until it's perpendicular to the floor.

Lower the weight and repeat. Once you've completed all of the prescribed repetitions, change positions and perform the exercise with your right arm.

Snatch-Grip Deadlift on Box

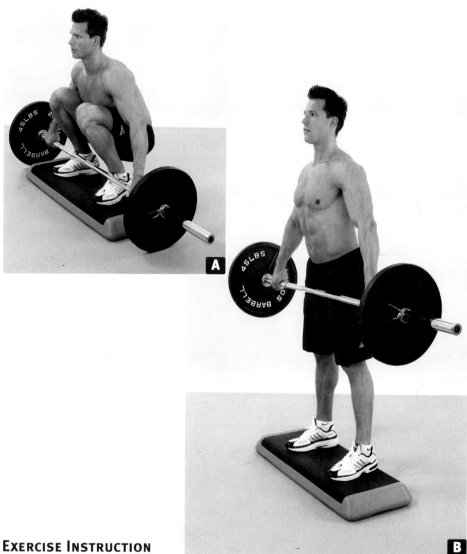

EXERCISE INSTRUCTION

(A) Set a loaded barbell on the floor and stand on a box facing it. (The box should be low enough that the barbell rises above your feet.) Squat down and grab it overhand, your hands about twice shoulder-width apart. Keep your back naturally arched.

(B) Without allowing your lower back to round, stand up with the barbell, pulling your shoulder blades back.

Slowly lower the bar to the starting position.

WORKOUT C
Incline Dip

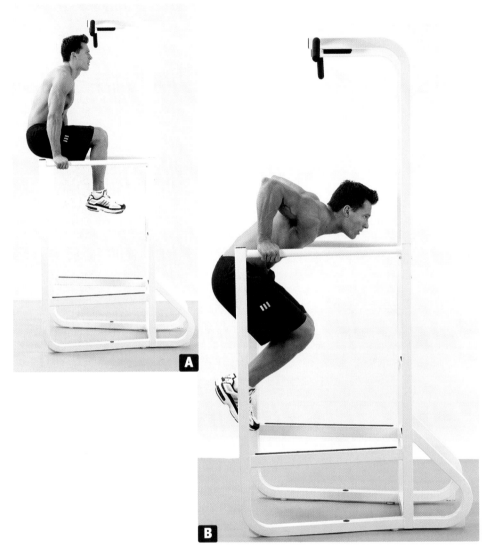

EXERCISE INSTRUCTION

(A) Grab the bars of a dip station and lift yourself so your arms are fully extended. Bend your hips and knees 90 degrees and hold them that way.

(B) Bend your elbows and slowly lower your body until your upper arms are at least parallel to the floor.

Pause, then push yourself back up to the starting position.

Incline Dumbbell Press

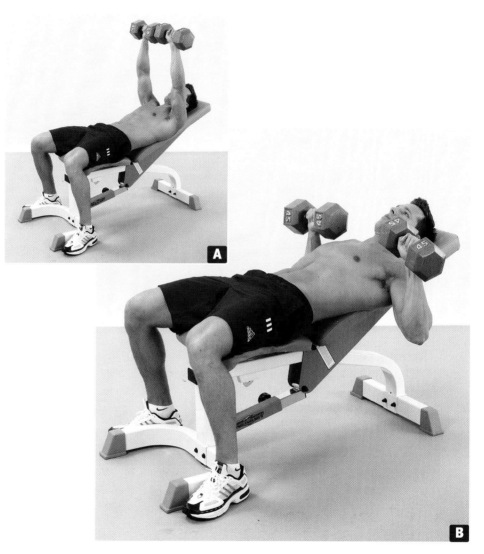

EXERCISE INSTRUCTION

(A) Grab a pair of dumbbells and lie on your back on a bench set to a low incline (15 to 30 degrees). Lift the dumbbells up at arm's length so they're over your chin, and hold them with your palms turned toward your feet so that your thumbs are facing each other.

(B) Slowly lower the weights to your upper chest, pause, then push them back up over your chin.

WORKOUT C

Swiss-ball Lying to Sitting Offset Dumbbell Curl

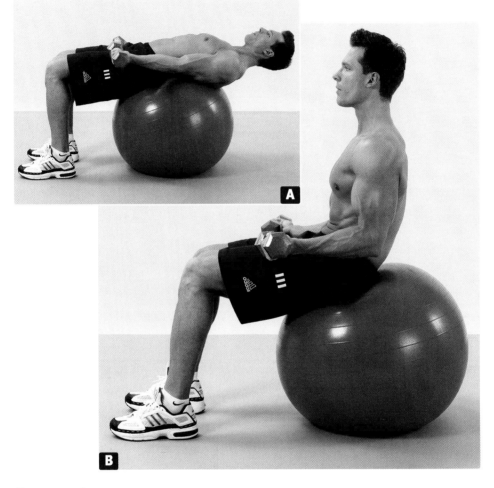

EXERCISE INSTRUCTION

(A) Grab a pair of dumbbells with an offset, underhand grip, so that your thumb is pressed against the outside head of the dumbbell. Lie on your middle and upper back on a Swiss-ball and keep your hips elevated so that your body forms a straight line from your knees to your shoulders. Hold your arms straight so that they're parallel to your body, your palms facing up.

(B) Raise your torso to a sitting position, keeping your forearms parallel to the floor, but bending your elbows so that your upper arms stay in line with your torso.

Reverse the movement to return to the starting position. That's one repetition.

Lying Triceps Extension to Close-Grip Bench Press

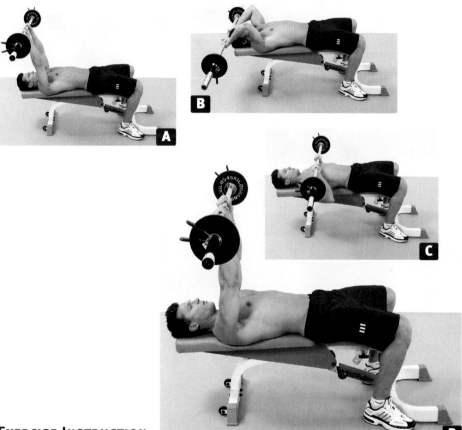

EXERCISE INSTRUCTION

(A) Grab a barbell and lie on your back on a bench. Hold the barbell above your forehead with an overhand grip, your hands about shoulder-width apart.

(B) Without moving your upper arms, lower the bar until your lower arms are almost perpendicular to the floor.

Pause, then raise the bar back to the starting position by straightening your arms.

Once you achieve technical failure, immediately (without resting) complete as many close-grip bench presses as you can by bending your elbows and lowering the weight to your chest **(C)**, then pushing it straight back up **(D)**.

When you achieve technical failure on the close-grip bench press, move on to the next exercise.

CHAPTER 11 ▶

Instant Answers:
Chest and Arms Specialization

THIS SUPPLEMENTAL Q AND A IS DESIGNED to answer common questions about this program, providing more details of how to execute the workouts, as well as additional explanation of many of the concepts presented throughout the book.

Why do we only do each workout for two weeks?

One main reason: Do too much for too long and you'll end up with no gains – or an injury. In this program, a high amount of "stress" is applied to specific tissues, energy systems and your central nervous system. Each has a finite rate of adaptability and tolerance. And the specialization phase is designed to progressively tax them to the max. It's sort of a kick in the pants in order to cause a quick jump in their rate of adaptability, accelerating gains in muscle size.

If you do it right, you should feel a little drained physically and ready for a change of pace by the end of the specialization program. Let's use an example to try to illustrate how this works. Picture your muscle as a bucket of water. The size of the bucket represents the size of your muscle. The water in the bucket represents your energy reserves and the materials that you can use for training, recovery and further growth. Each workout in a training program – like the Maximum Muscle Workouts – will dip a little bit of water out of the bucket. Between each workout, you rest and eat and the bucket adapts in proportion to the amount of water removed, growing a little bigger. This allows it to hold more water. In other words, the muscle increases in size and gains the capacity to do more work.

The specialization program takes a much bigger dip of water out of the bucket than the other workouts in this book. So the bucket gets bigger faster (as do your muscles). But because of the increased frequency and utilization of different training methods in this plan, you most likely won't be able to fully recover between each workout. That means you won't be able to replace all of the water you dipped out between workouts.

As you can probably guess, if this process continues for too long, there will eventually be little or no water left in the bucket. This is the point where things start to break down and progress stops, goes backward or you get hurt due to a lack of recuperative capacity. So it's important not to do a specialization phase too long.

What type of training should I do after the specialization cycle?

As you can see from the explanation above, the specialization program can be quite stressful. The biggest mistake would be to try to do another form of intensive training. Our best suggestion is to resume a less intensive program, much like the work capacity program in Chapter 3 or the first three weeks (phase 1) of the Maximum Muscle phase.

What are the reasons for the isometric bench press, static curl and static lying triceps extension? What do the "pauses" do?

There are actually a few reasons. Isometric or static contractions are muscle contractions against resistance but without movement – like pushing against a concrete wall or holding weights in a stretched position. Since most guys rarely perform prolonged isometrics, they are a novel stimulus to your muscles that can accelerate gains in size and strength faster.

A bonus feature is that isometric training can strengthen your connective tissues. That's because heavy loads on the connective tissue directly increase the amount of protein in the tendon, making it stronger and more injury-resistant. The sustained contractions also increase the accumulation of lactic acid in the muscles, which will promote a toughening of the sheath that surrounds the tendon. In addition, isometrics can increase the stiffness of tissues. That means the tendons can handle greater loads, increasing your potential to gain strength faster.

Why do we only do one repetition of the three-stop decline triceps extension?

If you set your weight appropriately so that

WHY DO WE LOWER THE WEIGHT FOR FIVE SECONDS ON SOME EXERCISES? HOW LONG SHOULD I TAKE TO LOWER THE WEIGHT ON THE OTHERS?

Lifting tempos – the speed at which you complete each repetition – have gotten a lot of attention in recent years. Because muscle tension is never constant throughout the full range of motion of a joint, specific tempo prescriptions are rarely a necessity. It's important to keep in mind that training adaptations do change when you alter the speed at which the weight is lifted. But it's rarely necessary to prescribe any more information than to lift a weight fast, slow, explosively or at a moderate pace. Most of the time, the amount of weight determines the speed that you lift the bar automatically. Ever try to lift a very heavy weight quickly? Try as you may, it won't move anywhere quickly (unless you drop it). So basically, let the weights determine the speed of movement while remaining in control of it at all times.

As for the five-second recommendation on some lifts, it's a communication tool for your understanding. We're trying to temporarily place greater emphasis on the lowering portion – known as the eccentric phase – of the lift. The reason: The eccentric phase has been shown to induce greater increases in size and strength than the concentric, or lifting phase. Does this mean we want to always perform slower eccentric contractions? Not really. It's simply another tool that we can use to stimulate faster gains. Again, we don't want to overuse it. Doing a slow eccentric all the time will eventually limit the amount of weight you can actually lift, since it speeds muscle fatigue.

The eccentric phase also has a unique quality of loading your muscles near the ends, where the tendons attach. This may provide a protection factor by increasing the durability of this area, which is prone to injury.

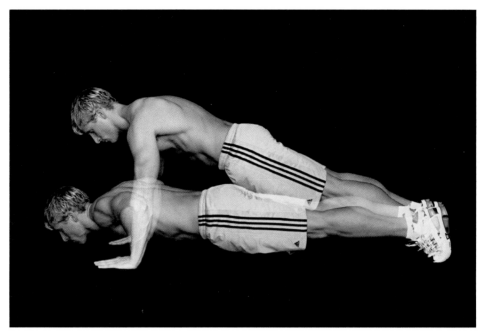

you can't hold beyond the prescribed duration of each stop, attempting a second "rep" at that weight for the prescribed durations will be virtually impossible. Also, consider that that the total duration of the "rep" actually lasts about as long as a set of about six to 10 reps. So your muscles are under tension for a similar amount of time as if you were doing a "normal" set, but they're stimulated in a different way.

Why do we use low reps and high reps on the same day? I thought you said that causes your body to try to adapt to too many stimuli?

We have several reasons in this case, but let's start with a favorite quote from top strength and conditioning coach Alwyn Cosgrove: "It's OK to break the rules as long as you know why you're breaking them." In other words, sometimes we have to deviate from the standards to achieve the training effect that we seek. This portion of the program is one of those times.

Think about this for a minute: Is your body the same as it was 12 weeks ago before you started this program? Absolutely not. Compared to your level of physical conditioning before beginning our workouts, your ability to activate your muscles is many times higher than before – you can lift more weight, you can train with a much higher level of mental and physical intensity and you can recover faster. The fact is that you're now a much more adaptable human being. So we can challenge your body a little more using different techniques. In the first couple of sets of each workout in the specialization phase, you'll stimulate your nervous and muscular systems heavily, which will cause you to hit technical failure. But you'll still have some energy to spare. So we've added in some lower-weight, higher-repetition sets to more fully train your energy systems. Remember, it's not something you want to do all the time because it's extremely taxing, but it works great to boost your results in a specialization phase.

Which diet do I follow in this phase?

For best results, go with the Maximum Muscle Diet. It'll ensure that you have all of the raw materials needed for muscle growth, as well as plenty of energy to perform the workouts.

CHAPTER 12 ▶

Instant Answers:
Troubleshooting and Preventive Maintenance

T**HIS SUPPLEMENTAL Q AND A IS DESIGNED** to answer common questions about this program, providing more details of how to execute the workouts, as well as additional explanation of many of the concepts presented throughout the book.

Should I "lock-out" when I lift?

Yes. We're not sure where the concept of not locking out the joints started, but it's been standard advice in many of the bodybuilding magazines over the past few years. The idea was probably to utilize the non-locking concept as a way to increase stimulus on the muscles and to protect the joints by keeping the muscles tensed for the entire movement. Truth be told, it may just work in reverse.

It's perfectly natural to lock-out your elbows and knees in daily activities and in exercises such as presses or squats. Not doing so actually limits your ability to produce strength when the knee or elbow is fully extended, which could be dangerous. If you can't produce force in the fully extended position, you're at risk for unprotected hyperextension (your joint overextends) resulting in a joint sprain or much worse.

Ever watch Olympic weightlifting? Those guys and gals have been locking out joints for years and have one of the lowest rates of injury in all of sports. Chances are that their joints are even less prone to injury than most folks walking down the street. Over time, the joints progressively adapt to the loading and the cartilage that covers the ends of the bones can actually get "tougher" and more resistant to injury.

There are a couple of tricks to doing it right, though. First rule: Always maintain control of the movement as you approach and achieve lock-out. In other words, don't slam the joint into a locked out position. Going too fast and losing control may result in extending too far or reaching a point of hyperextension, which is a great way to make your orthopedic surgeon a rich man. For those of you who naturally have the extra joint flexibility to hyperextend your joints – that is, you're "double jointed" – don't venture into that hyperextended region under load. You don't have the necessary muscular support in that range of motion. Practice achieving full extension but nothing more.

Second rule: Never relax in the extended, locked-out position. Remember, we want to teach the muscles to be active at this point. It's tempting to rest on the joint itself and take a breather, but resist the urge. Choosing to do so may result in an injury. So always keep your muscle contracted when your joints are locked.

Do I need to stretch?

Maybe. Flexibility is a personalized issue. Some people are very flexible and may never need to worry about changes in their flexibility. Others develop a great deal of increased tissue stiffness that contributes to greater strength levels, but can limit dynamic movement such as those during sports. With that in mind, consider the following principles to promote optimal flexibility.

A. Perform strength training throughout the full, safe, pain-free range of motion. This is actually one of the best ways to develop active flexibility. By performing exercises through a full range of motion, the connective tissues progressively adapt to necessary lengths, and strength is developed throughout the entire movement. This promotes a quality of injury protection at the end range of motion where most injuries occur.

B. Develop strength on all sides of the joints. In other words, complement every push exercise (press) with a pull (row). Many flexibility issues can be traced back to ill-designed pro-

---

MY SHOULDERS HURT WHEN I BENCH. WHAT SHOULD I DO?

The shoulder may be the most complicated joint in the entire body. There are so many influences that it would be impossible to determine any single cause in a book such as this. However, we can offer some basic concepts that may be helpful.

A. Posture affects shoulder function. Remember when your mom told you to sit up straight? She was right! Posture in which the back is rounded forward, the shoulders are rounded forward and the head shifts forward in a slouched position will predispose an individual to shoulder pain and potential injury. Get an assessment by a qualified health or fitness professional if you have any concerns in this area. (Stand sideways with a relaxed, natural posture and look at yourself in the mirror.) It could save you a lifetime of pain.

B. Strive for balanced strength between the front and the back of the shoulder. For every push exercise like a bench press, be sure to include a pulling exercise, like some form of rowing. Insufficient strength on one side of the joint will alter the way that the joint functions during exercise and activities of daily living. Over time, the joint will experience wear and tear that can result in pain or some form of permanent injury.

C. Technique, technique, technique. One of the most common reasons for shoulder pain during pressing exercises is simply poor form. During a bench press, the shoulders should be in a retracted (squeezed together) and depressed (pushed down) position. Allowing the shoulders to move upward away from the bench or shrugged up toward the ears places them in a less than ideal or unstable position and can overload the delicate connective tissues that passively stabilize the shoulder joint.

D. Don't overdo it. Another common technical issue is attempting to extend the set too far by performing beyond your capabilities in achieving muscular failure. It is quite common to see programs that emphasize continuing a set until no further repetitions can be performed, known as complete failure. In this program we have circumvented that issue by only continuing sets to a point of technical failure. Following the guidelines for technical failure as presented in Chapter 1 will go a long way in preventing injuries, while ensuring faster progress.

grams that neglect training the joints from multiple angles. As you work through this program, you'll see that that the workouts follow this principle quite nicely.

C. Perform dynamic movements at a variety of speeds and through an increasing range of movement without pain. You'll notice that your warm-ups consist primarily of active movements. By progressively increasing the range of movement and the speed of movement, the part of the nervous system which controls muscle extensibility adapts to allow the joints to move through a greater range of movement. So in your warm-ups, concentrate on lowering your body a little deeper each time you do the overhead squat, the squat, the good morning, the lunge and the Romanian deadlift.

Bottom line: If you're following the workouts as they're prescribed in this book, you're already doing a great deal of flexibility training. Unfortunately, due to individualized differences, you may need further flexibility training for optimal function. If you have any question as to whether stretching would be helpful, consult with a local health or fitness professional who is trained to assess your flexibility.

My heels come off the floor when I squat. Is that OK?

No. This is usually the result of a flexibility issue somewhere in the hip or ankle. Typically, most fitness professionals will conduct a full lower body assessment to determine the tight areas and then prescribe the appropriate flexibility program to address the tightness.

We have a better way. It takes a bit of patience and persistence, but it's extremely effective. Here's how it works: To prevent the heels from rising, widen your squat stance and point your toes outward about 30 degrees or so. The width of your stance and amount of "toe-out" will vary based on your flexibility, but it should be wide enough that you maintain the optimal posture throughout your set. (Optimal squat posture, in most cases, is with your torso in a fairly upright position with your lower back naturally arched for the entire movement.) This will allow you to perform the movement while keeping your heels flat. If they still rise slightly, just lower your body to the point at which they start to elevate. Each workout, try to lower a little farther. As you gain flexibility by performing squats through the full available range of motion, progressively narrow your stance and reduce your toe-out until you reach your desired squat stance.

My wrists hurt when I do push-ups and bench presses. Anything I can do?

Of course. If your wrists hurt when doing push-ups, it's probably an issue of a lack of wrist extension flexibility. (That is, the ability to extend your hand backward.) You can temporarily relieve the pain by performing your push-ups while holding dumbbells on the floor (not for the dynamic push-ups though!) or by doing push-ups on your fist (make sure to pad the floor). This helps to keep your wrists straight – maintaining a more "neutral" alignment of the wrist joint – and will relieve the pain. You may also want to regularly perform a few repetitions of regular pushups to encourage the development of increased wrist extension. Much like the squat example above, the wrists will slowly adapt and increase flexibility over time if trained consistently.

Wrist pain during the bench press is somewhat related, but usually includes a small technical issue. When grasping the bar for a bench press, the fingers and thumb should be wrapped firmly and fully around the bar, with the bar positioned on the heel of the hand (bottom of the palm). This distributes the load straight through the wrist joint in a neutral position. Think of it as keeping your wrists straight. Many guys make the mistake of allowing the bar to rest toward the pads of their palm near their fingers (around the area where calluses occur), which forces the wrist into an extreme extension or hyperextension of the wrist joint.

How do I keep from rounding my back when I deadlift?

Two ways: Practice and proper loading. During a deadlift, your spine should maintain what's called the neutral position. This is the same position that the spine is in when you stand up as tall as possible. In other words, your lower back is naturally arched. Rather than bending forward to perform the deadlift by rounding the spine, the bend actually comes from your hips. Your torso will incline forward when the bar is closer to the floor, but the same neutral position of the spine (naturally arched lower back) is maintained throughout the lift. So go through a mental checklist before you perform the movement. It may even help to look at your profile in the mirror before you lift. Adjust your posture if your back is rounded. Pulling your shoulders back, sticking your chest out and dropping your hips lower will help you achieve the correct body position.

The other cause of a rounded back during a deadlift is simply using the wrong load. Maybe it's the testosterone or the competitive nature of most guys, but using too much weight too soon is a sure trip to the spine doctor. The optimal load for the deadlift is one that allows you to maintain the neutral spinal position discussed above. If you can't maintain it throughout the full set, the set is over and you'll need to reduce the weight. (Remember technical failure?)

Is it OK to use lifting straps? What about gloves?

We don't usually recommend either, but occasional use of lifting straps may be OK when used judiciously. Straps may allow you to lift a little more weight or do an extra repetition or two due to weakness in the grip, but in the long run, they're probably not advantageous. Grip strength is a limiting factor in many exercises – even those you wouldn't suspect. For instance, a stronger grip will increase the number of chin-ups you can do and the number of curls you can do and the number of presses you can do. Try this quick test: Make a fist. Now make it tighter. And tighter. And even tighter. What happened? Did you feel how more and more muscle began to contract the tighter you made your fist? (Sometimes even

> Overuse of assistive devices like lifting straps doesn't allow the progressive increase in grip strength as going with a 'naked' grip does. **Save the straps** for your hardest sets

your jaw muscles will contract.) The same thing will happen as you increase your grip strength. You'll actually be able to increase the amount of stimulation your nervous system sends to your muscles. So they'll contract harder, which will transfer to your other exercises.

Our point: Overuse of assistive devices like lifting straps doesn't allow the progressive increase in grip strength as going with a "naked" grip does. Save the straps for your hardest sets where your grip may be a limiting factor and eventually try to eliminate their use entirely.

Weightlifting gloves are for hand models and women.

Should I wear a weight belt?

According to Dr. Stuart McGill, the world's foremost authority on the spine, the effect of a lifting belt is minimal as long as you maintain a neutral spine. (Sound familiar?) McGill submits that belts are only of significant benefit when lifting is performed with improper mechanics. Since we have gone to great lengths to emphasize the use of proper technique and proper loading throughout this program, the use of a weight lifting belt is not necessary.